Healthy Idol!

Trisha Stewart

Healthy Idol!

The Essential Guide to Eat Right, Avoid Excess, Get in Shape, Look Fabulous and Cope with Life: for Healthy Idols everywhere!

By Trisha Stewart

Healthy Idol

©2008 by Trisha Stewart

No portion of this book may be duplicated, copied, or used in any manner without expressed written consent of The Performance Marketing Group or Trisha Stewart under penalty of law.

Visit us on the web at:

www.HealthyIdol.com
www.TrishaStewart.com
www.ChristinMcdowell.com

ISBN 978-0-9816846-0-4

Other books by Trisha Stewart include:

    Healthy Tart
    Healthy Dude Book (September 2008)
    Healthy Bunch Cookbook (September 2008)

Trisha Stewart

Dedications

This book is dedicated to Luke, my eldest Grandson, now 18. He has taught me so many life lessons and now is finally going to listen to me!

Healthy Idol

Acknowledgements

My thanks to Mavis, Chris and the team as a whole. Young people are an incredibly important aspect of our society and I hope this book contributes in some way towards their development.

"If I said to most of the people who auditioned, 'Good job, awesome, well done,' it would have made me actually look and feel ridiculous. It's quite obvious most of the people who turned up for this audition were hopeless."

Simon Cowell

Contents

Preface	8
(1) So you wanna be a Healthy Idol?	10
• Dream Big	
• Set SMART Goals	
(2) Image is Everything...the RIGHT Image that is	20
• Look good, feel good, do good	
• You determine the meaning of success	
(3) Eating	33
• What, When & How Much	
• Fast Food...Friend or Foe?	
• Cool substitutes for Junk Food	
(4) Exercise	64
• There are no Idle Idols	
• Movin' it in style (be fit & Stylin')	
• Takin' it to the streets (get outside)	
(5) Everything Else	77
• Sex, Drugs & Rock n' Roll	
• Skin deep (caring for the outside package)	
(6) Obstacles	96
• Peer Pressure	
• Role Models...or the lack thereof	
• Stress, Fear & Loathing	
(7) Get it right...get support	109
• Make the right choices	

- Have a Plan B
- Don't go it alone

Idol Facts

Fact File A - The Future	123
Fact File B - Shopping List	125
Fact File C - Juices, Smoothies & Recipes	130
Fact File D - Fast Food	147
Fact File E - Drugs	156
Fact File F - Sexually Transmitted Diseases	165
Fact File G - Resources	172
Fact File H - THE GLYCAEMIC INDEX	174

Trisha Stewart

Healthy Idol

Preface

There is a phenomenon that has captivated the attention of the world's TV audience. Around the world, thousands upon thousands of kids from literally toddlers with proud parents through twenty-something year-olds with hopeful dreams line the streets to audition for the ubiquitous talent show. And, of course, the mother of all talent shows is the **American Idol / Pop Idol** franchise. **American Idol** has launched the careers of superstars like Kelly Clarkson and Carrie Underwood, as well as many other contestants who never made it to the actual 'Idol' finals. In the UK previously complete unknowns including Will Young, Paul Potts and the group Girls Aloud have skyrocketed into spectacular careers as a result of these talent shows.

This global sensation shows that so many of us want to achieve something special. We have a spark inside us and strive for our 15 minutes of fame. I am truly amazed by the human spirit and heartened by the raw talent, but too often devastated by the rate at which some of these gems burn so brightly only to fall so hard. It seems few of our talented youngsters are prepared for that journey or indeed for the consequences of that success.

Every time you watch the TV, read a magazine or surf the web, there appears to be another case of some young star heading for rehab, overdosing (on legal or illegal drugs), being charged with

Healthy Idol

drunken driving or on the verge of starvation. How can these talented young people go so far astray so quickly?

And it's not just in the field of entertainment. Young people in every walk of life are trying to better themselves and strive towards a brighter future. But there are obstacles along the way that many are unprepared for - stress, image/weight issues, peer pressure, bullying, drugs, alcohol abuse, depression and more.

That's why I decided to write this book as an easy-to-read and easy-to-understand guide providing alternatives to those negative paths. Let me say right now that this book is not about being squeaky clean or perfect! It's about how to reach for those lofty heights and make the right choices along the way. I want my readers to recognize the difference between assistance and exploitation, friends and social climbers, a few drinks and a binge. I want them to understand that the way to be at the top of their game is to be healthy - physically, mentally and emotionally.

Look, we're not all going to become an **American Idol**, but can dream...and given the right life choices, dedication and motivation, we can achieve the best that life has to offer us. This book is for anyone that wants to achieve something special and not get burned in the process. It is written primarily with younger people in mind but the advice and examples I offer are just as valid no matter who you are. So dream big and go for it...the **Healthy Idol** way!

Trisha Stewart - May 2008

Chapter 1

SO YOU WANNA BE A HEALTHY IDOL?

"If you dream and you believe, you can do it."
Sean P. Diddy Combs

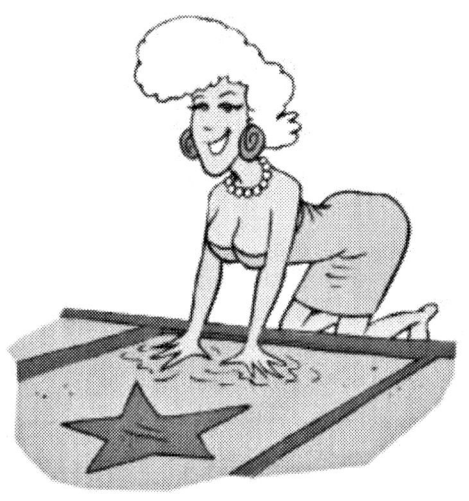

Admit it...even if just to yourself for right now. You want to be famous! Its okay...lots of people dream of being famous. Deep down we all want our 15 minutes of fame...the chance to stand in the spotlight, hear the applause and be adored for doing something really well. Think about it. Any time you've received recognition for something you did well, you loved it. Its human nature to want to be appreciated...and being appreciated is a good thing. And, there are some of us that truly crave that recognition and are drawn to activities and careers that will feed that craving...the performing arts (acting, singing, dancing), sports (baseball, basketball, football), writing, painting...the list goes on.

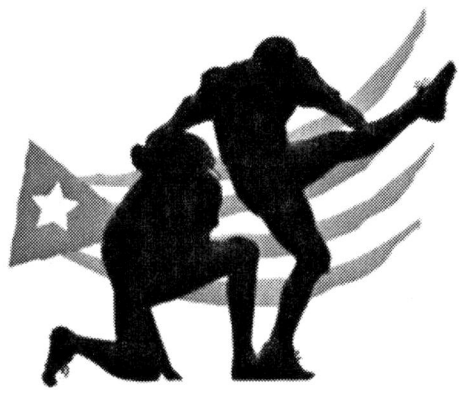

If it weren't the case...why would the most popular shows on television be talent competitions? *American Idol, You've Got Talent, Dancing with the Stars*...all top-rated shows that we not only watch, but talk about between episodes and hope to someday have the chance to appear on ourselves. If you're reading this book, I'm betting you are one of those people...you've got dreams and ambitions of fame, fortune, celebrity. You're ready for the big time and you're chances of making it are good. Why? Because you're smarter than a lot of other young people who just wish it would happen. You've decided to take action...go after your dreams and do it the right way...the healthy way. That's what *Healthy Idol* is all about. This book will help you set goals and work towards reaching your "Idol" ambitions – whatever they may be, while helping you stay healthy inside and out. In other words, to truly be a *Healthy Idol* you need to take care of your talent, your body and your mind. Well, I'm here to help.

Dream Big

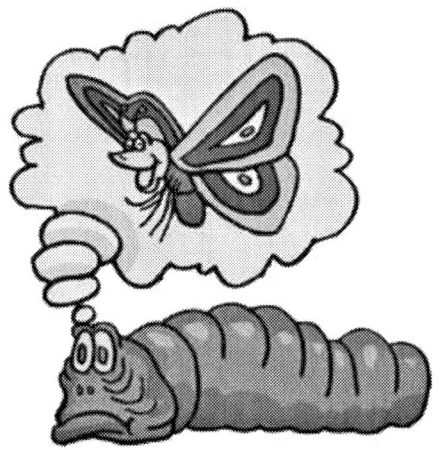

The first thing you need to do is set your sights on your goal. Now is not the time to hold back…go for it and reach high! What's the most amazing goal you can imagine? Is it performing on Broadway? Performing at Carnegie Hall? Singing to a sold-out crowd? Making it to the World Series? Writing a bestselling novel?

Whatever your passion…your talent…your skill…imagine how far you can take it and what you'd like to accomplish. It's more than just a vague idea. I want you to visualize yourself in that setting. Right now, I want you to sit somewhere quiet and comfortable. Close your eyes and take a deep breath. Forget about everything except your goal. Don't worry about what happened earlier in the day...or what you have to do later. Just think about the ultimate reward of your dream. Are you accepting an award? Giving an interview? Attending a premier? Whatever it is, I want you to see every detail. Picture everything around you. Where are you? What does the stage, studio or red carpet walk look like? What you're wearing? Who's there with you? How do you feel? What do you hear? What do you see around you?

Did you do it? I hope so, because it works! You see the biggest part of making any dream a reality is first making it real in your mind. Did you know that Jim Carrey used to head up into the Hollywood hills and look down over Los Angeles? There he would visualize his own dreams of making it as an actor...right down to the suit he was wearing at the award show.

This was all BEFORE he'd "made it". Did it work? Well, now he earns around $20 MILLION per movie...that's right $20 MILLON. So, yes I'd say it worked, wouldn't you? And, if you can't see yourself in that situation...then it's likely never going to happen! Jim Carrey knew that...and now, so do you. So, start imagining that place you want to end up right now. The more details you can see and visualize the more real it will become to you. Make it real in your mind and then make it real in your life!

So, you've got the detailed vision and now you can just sit back and wait for it to happen, right? Of course not! You know that just imagining your dreams coming true won't make them happen. It takes a lot of hard work and determination. And, everyone who DOES make it...makes their dreams come true...they all have something in common. They have all worked hard to hone their talent, persevered through challenges and kept on going.

So – here's your quick dose of reality, a little cold water in your face: If you're not going to work hard then you're never going to achieve your dreams! There, I said it. So you need to decide right now if you're willing to do the work. You're ready aren't you? I knew it! I could tell you were one of the special, determined, driven talented ones. You can visualize it all becoming a reality and you're ready to hit the ground running, right? Okay, then...drum roll please... welcome to the world of *Healthy Idols!* Let's get started!!

"Don't compromise yourself. You are all you've got."
Janis Joplin

Once you have your vision...you need to set short and long term goals to help you achieve it...steps to mark your progress along the way. If you don't have any way to measure your success, growth and improvement...you won't have any way to you're heading in the right direction and staying on track.

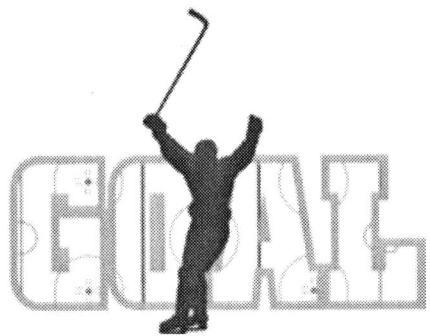

Your goals are much more specific than your vision. Your vision may be to get a recording contract, but your goals are the way you get closer to that contract...one accomplishment at a time. So, what are some specific goals for you?

- Find a voice coach and take singing lessons
- Audition for a local play
- Improve your basketball free throws
- Get some headshot photographs taken
- Lose some weight and become more fit
- Tryout for a sports team
- Take an acting class
- Learn to play a musical instrument

Now, setting goals is one thing. Making sure you set good goals that help you improve yourself, keep you on track and yet won't be so hard to reach is another matter! So what you should do is to make your goals **S.M.A.R.T. goals**. This is a system of setting goals that help ensure you can actually achieve them. So, let's take a look at what **S.M.A.R.T. goals** are:

Specific: *Don't say, "I want to be a singer." Instead say, "I want to be singing with a local band in six months." That way it's very easy for you to see how much you're improving and you'll feel great when you get there.*

Measurable: *Give yourself something you can truly measure. If your goal is to get headshot photographs taken, there are steps you can break down: Get a list of quality photographers, meet with them, view their portfolio, get an estimate of what it will cost, save the money, set the appointment. You can check off each piece as you get it done and measure how close you're getting.*

Attainable: *Can you make this happen? Do you have the skills, resources, knowledge and desire to reach your goal? Can you get those needed things? If you want to be a singer, but aren't sure if you can carry a tune, then find a voice coach that will give you an honest assessment of your skills. From there you'll know how to adjust your vision.*

Realistic: *This is really up to you...if you work at this, can it happen? An unrealistic goal would be "I'm going to get a* recording contract in the next six months!" Not only is it unrealistic, but you'll be setting yourself up for frustration and disappointment when it doesn't happen. Not sure about what's unrealistic and what's a good challenge? Share your goals with someone you trust for some support and feedback.

Timely: *Having a timetable attached is the best way to keep on track. Make sure you have target dates of when you want to accomplish and meet your different goals. If you don't have an end-date in mind, there's no incentive to get started. If there's a date to try out for the team or audition for a play then you've got a built in timeframe right there!*

We've made it even easier for you to set your goals. With the S.M.A.R.T. tips in mind...you can complete the "FUTURE WHEEL" worksheet from **Fact File** A (at the end of the book). This is something you can copy and stick up on the wall or bathroom mirror to remind yourself of where you're headed!

Remember that your goals are a way for you to meet your big dream...your vision. But you may need to adjust your goals along the way...or even make new and different ones. As long as your goals are getting you closer to your big dream, you're heading in the right direction.

Keeping you and your goals healthy

Keep in mind that maintaining or improving your health needs to be one of your most important goals! Whether you're going after something physical like playing sports or something artistic like singing...if you're not in the best health you can be you won't have the stamina and strength to accomplish your dream. Trying to determine what is healthy these days, especially looking at many so called celebrity role-models might just be your biggest challenge. But, that's where *Healthy Idol* can help. This entire book is focused on giving you the truth about eating, exercise and everything else. Here are some of the key points you'll learn:

1. The FOUR Foundation Stones to Build the Best YOU!
2. What to eat, how much to eat and when to eat it
3. The REAL truth about fast food
4. How to get fit fast...without joining a gym
5. What drugs are REALLY doing to your mind and body
6. How to recognize, face and overcome obstacles to your dream
7. Tips for making the right choices for YOU
8. Why you need a Team to support you along the way (and how to build it)

"The worst crime is faking it."
Kurt Cobain

You've got your vision, you've set some goals and you're ready to put them into action. **Healthy Idol** has the steps, truth and

Healthy Idol

tips you need to make your dream a reality. Are you ready to take each step, fight the good fight and stick with it? Great, because guess what? Tomorrow is coming no matter what, so I want to make sure it gets you one day closer to your dream!

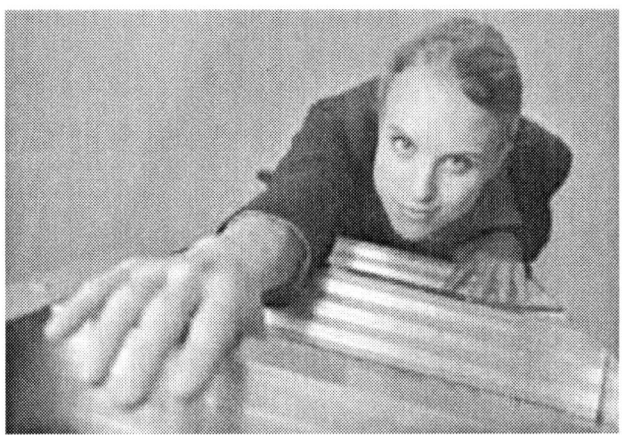

Chapter 2

IMAGE IS EVERYTHING...THE RIGHT IMAGE THAT IS

"Years ago I asked my dad for a boob job, but he said it would cheapen my image."
Paris Hilton

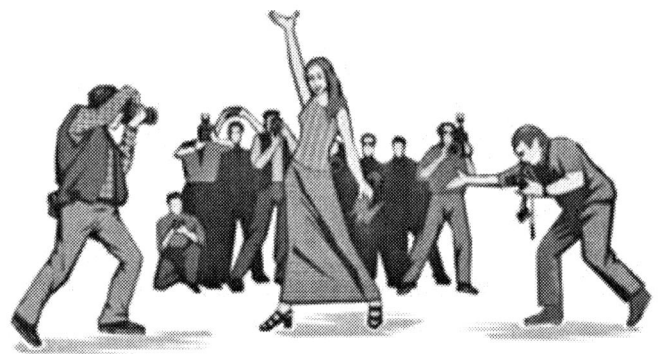

If image weren't important, how could so many people be famous for doing absolutely nothing but being who they are and presenting that certain, desired image? Don't believe me? Take our quotable gal, Paris Hilton...what does she do? She's Paris, that's what. Love her or not...she's famous for her image.

Things that make you go...hmmmmm! So, no matter what we think about celebrity and fame...image is a big part of it all. From first impressions to lasting ones, what people think about us has an impact. And, if you're thinking about being a Healthy Idol, what other people think about you can make or break you.

Bottom line...there's a lot of pressure to measure up to what 'others' think you should be or represent! Have you been thinking about what you want your image to be? How will you develop it? Is it the right one?

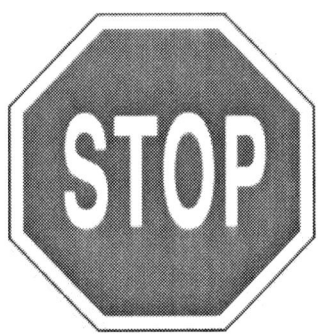

Before you get all worked up about your image...how you should look, what you should wear...there's something very important to know and remember. Image is more than just the outside package...it's about how you present yourself and how you feel about yourself. The right image is about creating a whole, complete, healthy, happy, focused person.

Look Good, Feel Good, Do Good

Sure, it all starts with how you look...so let's get started. Looking your best is really about the basics. I call them the Four Foundation Stones to building the best you!

The Four Foundation Stones

1. Eating Right (and the right amount)
2. Exercising
3. Drinking Enough Water
4. Getting Enough Rest

EATING RIGHT

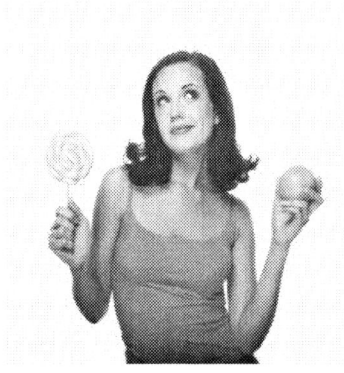

I've put lots of information in this book about how to eat right, what to avoid and how to deal with tough situations like fast food restaurants and snacking. I've even included a simple, effective 24-hour 'recovery' for when you do give in to the burgers, fries and junk. Plus, there are ideas for healthy snacks so you can have good-for-you options when you're on the go. That means it will be easier for you to stay on track and triumph over temptations.

Healthy Idol

EXERCISE

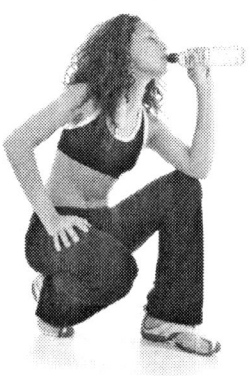

And, chances are if you're under 20, you probably spend a lot of time on the computer...more time than you do exercising and moving. Whether you're checking out your MySpace page, playing the latest online video game or just surfing the net...that's just not enough action to get your body Healthy Idol fit.

Now, I realize that kids today often have busier schedules than their parents...but carving out time for physical activity is a TOP TEN priority (along with other things that will help you reach and achieve your Healthy Idol goal). That's why I worked with my fitness expert, Christin McDowell, on ways to get you back in gear on taking care of your body. From working out without a gym to how to get fit fast...we've got some great ways for you to get up, get in shape AND have fun while you do it.

And remember to **GET YOUR EIGHTS**!

That's eight 8-ounce glasses of water a day and eight hours sleep.

Your specific needs may vary, but if you haven't at a minimum been 'getting your eights'...then it's a great starting point. But keep in mind everyone is a bit different and therefore, obviously, your personal requirements may vary.

DRINKING ENOUGH WATER

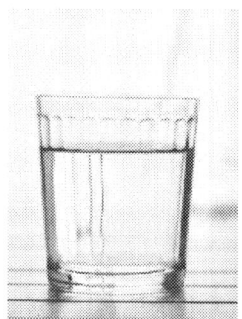

Let's look at how much water you should drink. The established average is eight 8-ounce glasses per day...because that's the average. And, since most people don't drink nearly enough water establishing an average helps you measure how you're doing. In getting more specific, your daily water intake should be half your body weight in ounces. So, if you weigh 120 pounds - that means 60 ounces of water (darn close to the 8 oz theory, which totals up to 64 ounces). But, if you weigh more, say 150...then you need to be working towards drinking 75 ounces of water per day. Of course, the actual amount you need to drink is not only based around your weight, but how active you are. If you're exercising, have a more physical job or live in an arid climate, you'll need to take in more liquids to stay hydrated, alert and healthy! Make sense? Great, now let's talk about sleep!

GETTING ENOUGH SLEEP

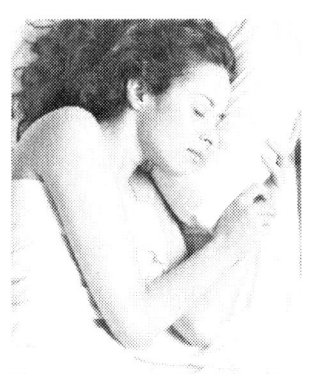

Do people really need eight hours of sleep? Well, like how much water your body needs, the amount of sleep you need varies too. For example, newborn babies can sleep and nap around 16-20 hours a day! They need that sleep as their bodies and brains are developing. But, we'd be hard pressed to get much done if we slept that much, right? Don't worry; you don't need that much sleep anymore.

The 'eight-hour' average is for most typical adults. However, teens and growing kids can require a bit more than that...up to 9.5 hours...especially as you go through puberty. Puberty is a growth period for your body and just like babies need extra hours, you will too for a few years. The biggest problem is that with your jam-packed schedule, you're probably not even getting eight hours of sleep. Studies show that many teens and young adults are actually sleep deprived.

You may not think missing a little sleep is a big deal...but it adds up. If you miss one hour of sleep every night for a week, it's like missing one full night of snoozing. Besides putting you in a grumpy mood, lack of sleep can decrease your attentiveness and short-term memory. And, let's not forget delayed response time and inconsistent performance. And, if you expect to be a Healthy Idol, you've GOT to be consistent.

One bad performance and you could lose a chance of a lifetime, right? If that's not enough to get you to a regular sleep schedule, think about this...sleep deprivation can cause driving accidents. In fact, more than half 'asleep-at-the-wheel' car accidents are caused by teens. **So, get some sleep!**

So, the **Four Foundation Stones to building the best you** probably make a lot of sense to you now. But, you're probably asking 'how does feeling good help my image?' Well, I'm glad you asked! Feeling good is not just about physically feeling good...it's about your self-esteem or confidence.

You may have heard it before, but if you want others to like you, you have to first like yourself. So, how do you do that? You make decisions and choices that you can live with for the long-term. It can be a challenge with all the pressure around to make bad choices. And, sometimes it's hard for young adults like you to think past the weekend...let alone five, ten or twenty years from now.

Often times what might be fun in the short-term can have long-term negative results. There are some obvious things that fall into that category – drugs, alcohol and sex all come to mind. I address the reality of these very things in **Chapter Five - *Everything Else***. I get that life can be difficult, and sometimes struggles and challenges can seem overwhelming... especially for teenagers. Sometimes those people you'd like to rely on to support and guide you are actually steering you in the wrong direction. That's why I walk with you through the reality of peer pressure, role models and other influences that can make it hard to stay on track in **Chapter Six - *Obstacles***.

When it comes right down to it...you're the one who has to make decisions for yourself...no one else can do it for you. So, focus on what's right for you. Next time you're stuck between Option A or Option B (Deal or No Deal) imagine this...which choice will make it easy for you to look at yourself in the mirror the next day...the day after that...the rest of your life?

What do I mean? "Looking yourself in the mirror" means you'll have to think about the long term effects of your decision...for you and for others. It will help you make choices that are right and healthy for you and do not hurt or harm others. That way you can smile back at your reflection; not just because of how you look, but because of how you feel.

Confidence shines through when you know you're doing the best you can for yourself. And, people who have that inner confidence or good self-esteem stand out from the crowd. For Healthy Idols, being outstanding...having that certain something...is vital.

"Mom always tells me to celebrate everyone's uniqueness.
I like the way that sounds."
Hilary Duff

Now, I'd like to take the idea of 'feel good' a bit further into 'do good.' While making right and healthy choices for yourself is a big part of developing a positive image, what you do for others completes the package.

Don't worry...I'm not telling you that you have to go out and save the world by ending hunger...it's much simpler than that. Start with how you treat your friends and family. You've heard the Golden Rule, right? Treat others the way you'd like to be treated. Maybe you don't think how you treat others matters too much, but let's take a look at some who've not been too kind.

Ever hear of Naomi Campbell? Russell Crowe? Both made headlines for their poor behavior towards others. Top model Naomi Campbell has even found her way into court because of abuse towards her personal assistants (yes, that's plural...she's got a reputation). And after Russell Crowe hurled a phone at a hotel employee he lost major good image points and had to go to great lengths to rebuild it (he's not really done yet).

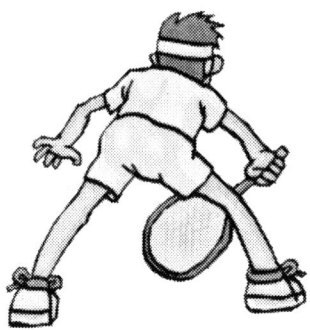

Think about this...tennis great John McEnroe had a major reputation as an ill-mannered, temper tantrum throwing athlete. Now he's regaining popularity by doing a series of commercials based on the fact that now he 'gets it' and treats people with respect. Bottom line...being nice is a good thing.

I'm not saying you're not already a nice, kind person...I'm sure you are. But just think about how you treat people, find ways to do good for others and you'll be building a solid, positive reputation. Reputation is just how others perceive and feel about your image. So, smile at people as you walk down your school hallways, and not just the cool kids...smile at everyone.

A couple of things will happen...people will smile back and you'll feel great. The better you feel, the more you'll smile and then you'll feel even better. Now imagine going from smiling to saying a few kind words or offering a helping hand. Just remember the Golden Rule and find ways to 'do good!'

You Determine the Meaning of Success

By now you've probably set your goals to reach your big dream...congratulations! If not...go to **Fact File A** right now and work on your Future Wheel! Been there, done that? Great! So, you're imagining being an Academy Award winning actor or a multi-platinum recording artist or a Broadway star...or something else that ignites a passion inside you.

Keep dreaming big, but realize that even if you don't attain that ultimate level you can still be a success. You may be the 'next big thing', but not everyone can be. Let me clarify that; I'm not saying you should stop trying to make your big dream come true. But every step you take along the way means you're successful. That's why you need to decide what being a success is...so you can feel good about whatever you accomplish.

Healthy Idol

You can be a success if you have a great garage band and have a great time playing for your friends at local parties. Getting a few parts at the local theater can still fulfill your need to perform and entertain a crowd. Plus, you'll want to develop your Plan B (see chapter 7 about that) so you'll always land on your feet. And, believe it or not, you may actually change your mind about going after your dream.

Maybe you'll decide singing isn't what you really want to do or playing sports is not how you want to make your living. That happens to people all the time...we always want to try something new or make a change on the path we've chosen. In other words, changing your mind is okay! It doesn't mean you've wasted time or been spinning your wheels. You've learned things along the way, gained some skills and bettered yourself. So, dream on and dream big. You may have what it takes to go all the way and I'm here to help you do it the healthy way. So, once you get on top...you can stay there.

"We've become so glorified in the movie-star system that it's become this artificial royalty. The truth is that we're circus clowns."
Nicolas Cage

Remember, the right image is a key step to your success...no matter what your goal. And, as I said at the beginning of this chapter...there's a lot of pressure to paint the right picture...be what other people expect you to be...and do it quickly. But, slow down. Remember that once you lock onto the right image for yourself, you need to be able to keep it up for the long haul.

So, avoid the quick fixes and fad approaches that you just can't keep up. Besides they're rarely, if ever, healthy options. Please, read the rest of this book to get the guidelines and tips you need to make long-term, good-for-you changes. You'll be on your way to developing the best you...someone you can live with and respect for a lifetime.

Healthy Idol

Chapter 3

EATING

*"Last time I ate was like two, three years ago...
I promise I will eat next week, swear to God."*
Nicole Ritchie

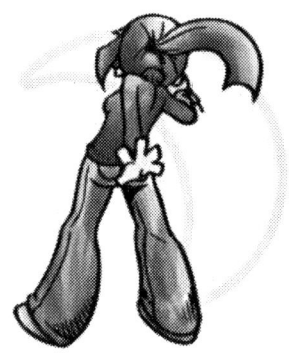

Sometimes I look at these beautiful, young people who seem to have it all and I just want to...give them a sandwich! I'm serious, it's clearly the one thing they don't seem to have handy. Yet, here's the wacky world we live in: by 2015 75% of adults and 24% of children and teens in America will be overweight or obese (according to researchers at the **Johns Hopkins Bloomberg School of Public Health**), but our standard of 'beauty' has shrunk to be a size ZERO! Is there no middle ground? Yes there is...and that's where Healthy Idols live.

So...here's a look into the world of eating: What, When & How Much!

What to Eat

It's really hard to figure out what you should or should not eat! There are so many opinions about what's good, what's bad, what's easy, what's cool, what's fun, what's safe and even what's environmentally or socially responsible to eat.

We are told that if we eat that type of food, or drink that special flavored water we will in fact be happier, smarter, cooler, sexier or more popular. We are even told we can make a difference in the world because every time we buy, they donate to a cause or charity. Now, let me say right here that I don't expect food manufactures to stop advertising, and I actually think big corporations should give back to communities and charities. But, there is so much conflicting advice it can be downright impossible to figure out the truth.

Don't think you get hit with lots of messages about food? Think about this...more than 34% of all the commercials shown during programs most kids watch are for convenience or fast foods. And 57% of food-related ads targeted toward adults focus on those same products. That's just on television... there's also advertising on the radio, online, on billboards...commercials are everywhere. You're bombarded by messages and they often contradict each other. How in the heck are you supposed to know what's best! Feeling hungry yet?

Did you know?	*The study by researchers at the University of Illinois at Urbana-Champaign is the first to explore the nutritional composition of foods advertised to children using Nutrition Facts labeling.*

What you need to remember is that food is fuel and you need to 'fill your tank' with foods that are good for you. Did you know that eating the wrong foods can cause you to be depressed? Seriously, your body chemistry alters according to what you put in your mouth! Not only does it affect your emotions, but eating the wrong foods can show in your skin, hair, nails and even bowel movements (you know - poo!) Yes, they are a normal function.

Working alongside the skin, kidneys and liver it's how our bodies eliminate waste and toxins. Remember that eating right is the *Foundation Stone #1* in building the best you. And, if you eat bad foods not only will you feel bad, but you'll have a weak foundation...one that won't be strong enough to support your journey towards *Healthy Idolness*.

Okay, after reading that you'll probably agree with my earlier comment that figuring out what to eat is a big challenge. And it will be if you try to gather your nutritional knowledge from advertising. But, it doesn't have to be that hard. In fact, I'm going to make it easy for you by giving you a list of the really good foods to incorporate into your daily life.

Simple though these foods may seem, they are the basis to a good diet. They're easy to find, easy to prepare, easy to eat and easy to dispose of anything that is not suitably edible. Real whole foods that come in their own packages, not wrapped in cardboard or plastic from the supermarket shelf or the drive thru.

So here are some very simple basics, you all know about but let's think about them in a different way

Fruits

- Enjoy all kinds of fruits. You can eat them whole or sliced and diced for snacking and salads. Drink them as juice or blend up your favorites into tasty smoothies. And, don't feel like you have to stick with the same fruits you always eat…be daring and try some star fruit, mango, kiwi, fresh figs or fresh dates…something else new and different.

Vegetables

- Okay, this might be a challenge if you're pretty 'anti-veggie' but try to keep an open mind. I know someone who used to think she HATED cooked vegetables until she had them lightly sautéed. What she really hated

Healthy Idol

were veggies boiled beyond flavor a
that's how they had been served to he
maybe you've never really been offe
way of vegetables...cooked or raw.

A good way to experiment with flavors is to try them grated or chopped raw, steamed lightly, sautéed or just plain boiled (but not over-boiled...remember my friend's experience). And, of course the least amount of cooking the more enzymes and other nutrients you'll get.

That's why juicing is a great way to get your daily requirement of vegetables. You can put so many different veggies in, add some apples for sweetness and you've got a tasty, healthy drink in minutes. You'll find some simple recipes for juicing in **Fact File C**.

Grains

- You're probably thinking about rice, right? Well, forget about that white fluffy stuff...all the good has been stripped away from that. I'm talking about real whole grains. They have great flavors and awesome chewy textures. Here again, you can try different types to see what you like. Sure, you can have brown and wild rice – that's a great place to start. But, sample some quinoa, millet, buckwheat and oats to add some variety.

eans or lentils

- These are a great source of healthy protein and carbohydrates. Think of Mexican style eating with re-fried beans, but stick with the vegetarian version to cut down on fats. There's also curried beans, bean salad and lentils, too. There are several types of lentils and many types of beans (check out the shopping list - **Fact File** B for a complete list). And, you can also try sprouting (to learn more about sprouting, check out my website at www.trishastewart.com or checkout some of my other books).

Nuts and seeds

- No they are NOT just for birds (and I'm talking more than just peanut butter here). Nuts and seeds are a great source of protein and essential fats. Plus they're perfect for snacking on the go as they're easy to carry with you. Try making some healthy alternatives to dairy butter or those awful soft margarines; nut butters are delicious, easy to make and add a different flavor to what you are going to eat. See the **Fact File**s for recipes.

This is just a brief introduction to what you need to get you going every day. And, I have created a detailed shopping list in **Fact File B** that you and your family can use so you'll be able to find all these goodies in your own cupboards. But, you can also find these types of foods when you're hanging out with your friends at your local juice and smoothie bars and whole food restaurants.

Yes, there are plenty of really healthy eating out places, check the internet for what is in your area, log into healthy cafe's or restaurants, Asian, Mexican whatever you like, keep away from the mass market restaurants they are actually expensive and will use a lot of chemicals. And, better still be a leader in the field and cook at home. I've included some fun recipes **(Fact File C)** you can whip up for your friends and family. Get cooking for them show them the healthy way forward...that tastes great!

Food Labels

Before I move on to *when* to eat...let's take a closer look at what you're actually eating. It's a good idea to know as much as you can about the food you're putting into your mouth. And, with so much processed and packaged food out there, that means you really need to understand food labels and the information they have.

Lets start with fresh food. Have you ever noticed a food label on a fresh piece of fruit, apart from where it came from? No! That's because there's nothing in fresh fruits and vegetables but the actual whole food and lots of good nutrition.

But, with any processed or packaged food, there are nutritional information labels that tell you everything from the serving size to how many calories (breaking that down into protein, carbohydrates and fats), to vitamin information and – of course – a complete list of ingredients.

How much you need and how we measure that is what I call a "work in progress." Scientists are continually improving their knowledge about the value of foods in response to our physiological requirements. And, what I need will be different from what you need…what you need will likely vary from what your friend needs. It all depends on a number of factors including age, sex, activity level, vitamin needs and more.

But, let's keep it simple. To be honest, I believe food labeling is there to warn you what NOT to eat. There are two fundamental parts to a food label – the ingredients and the nutrional information. So, when you look at a label…if there are ingredients listed that don't sound like food (or you can't pronounce them) chances are you shouldn't eat it. And, when you study the nutrional information…you can see if it's too high in calories, fat or sugars to be good for you.

The U.S. Food and Drug Administration's website has an excellent description of food labels and what you should be looking out for.

Healthy Idol

I will briefly describe the key facts on a typical food label but for a more comprehensive description, you should visit the FDA website at the following location:

www.cfsan.fda.gov/~dms/foodlab.html

Take a typical food label - it looks something like this:

Sample label for Macaroni & Cheese

Nutrition Facts

Serving Size 1 cup (228g)
Servings Per Container 2

Amount Per Serving

Calories 250   Calories from Fat 110

	% Daily Value*
Total Fat 12g	18%
Saturated Fat 3g	15%
Trans Fat 3g	
Cholesterol 30mg	10%
Sodium 470mg	20%
Total Carbohydrate 31g	10%
Dietary Fiber 0g	0%
Sugars 5g	
Protein 5g	
Vitamin A	4%
Vitamin C	2%
Calcium	20%
Iron	4%

* Percent Daily Values are based on a 2,000 calorie diet. Your Daily Values may be higher or lower depending on your calorie needs.

		Calories:	2,000	2,500
Total Fat		Less than	65g	80g
Sat Fat		Less than	20g	25g
Cholesterol		Less than	300mg	300mg
Sodium		Less than	2,400mg	2,400mg
Total Carbohydrate			300g	375g
Dietary Fiber			25g	30g

Here's a quick rundown of facts about calories, protein, fats, carbohyrdates, sodium and fiber...the things that 'make up' the food you eat.

Calories - this is the amount of food energy the item contains

- Helpful if you want to know how many calories to eat during the day - this will depend on whether or not you are on a weight reducing diet or if you are participating in sport - other than that there are only so many calories you need during the day to stay alive! Under "normal" circumstances we need around 2000 - 2500 calories daily, which of course need to come from a natural source. And, believe it or not, a burger and fries three times a day is NOT the best option for your calories. I know... SHOCK! HORROR! WHO KNEW?!

Protein - this means the amount of protein available in the product

- Protein can be from an animal or vegetable source and it is the build and repair part of the diet. We need it for every body cell. The RDA (recommended daily amount) as set out by the government is, in my opinion, far in excess of what we actually need. I know, of course, that people love to eat their meat, cheese, dairy and fish, etc. But with increased protein comes an increase in saturated fats...and that's not good at all. In reality, we only need around 5-6% of our diet to be protein. It doesn't hurt to eat more, but make sure anything in excess of that 5-6% is a non-animal sort such as nuts, seeds, grains and beans.

Fats - you will see two values here - 'total' and 'saturated' (and on this label even trans fats, which is a chemically altered processs to an unsaturated fat to make it more saturated. Increasing the level of bad cholesterol LDL and as many young people eat this stuff, heart disease is on the increase in the younger age group)

- It's really the percentage of total fat that comes from saturated fat that you need to watch. Fat can be from animal or vegetable origin. Take note that coconut and palm oil is a saturated fat but the main source is usually of animal origin. So, watch the saturated fats!!!

Carbohydrates - again you will see two values here a "total" and "sugars"

- Counting or watching your 'carb' intake can be very tricky. If you are diabetic or on a low carb diet you really need to know about carbs, and I don't just mean total carbs, but whether they are complex carbs or simple sugar carbs. You're looking for where things fall on the Glyceamic Index (GI) - See **Fact File** H. This is where the ingredients list comes in handy. You can see if the sugars are coming from a vegetable or fruit source or if they are from grains, high fructose corn syrup or other sugars (dextrose, maltodextrin, etc). Complex carbohydrates from whole grains, beans, lentils and vegetables are healthy. But, simple sugar carbohydrates are dangerous if you're diabetic and they contain little, if any, food value for the body.

Sodium (sodium chloride is salt)

- This will just show the amount of grams of sodium – but it could be naturally available in the foods or added. You need to avoid anything added...so here again, the ingredients are important. Keep to a maximum of 1 teaspoon daily. And, that can be especially hard if you're eating things like fast food, chips, breakfast cereals. And, even healthy foods sometimes contain too much sodium.

Fiber

- Again the ingredients list is useful as there will be fiber available from vegetable, fruit, grain, bean or other cereals. You generally can't over eat on fiber and most people don't eat enough.

Okay...so reading the labels on EVERY food item you eat from morning cereal to late night snack not only sounds a bit daunting, but BORING! Don't you think? So, save yourself the hassles and eat more natural and whole foods. No labels to read, remember? All you have to do is choose from a good range of foods to include complex carbs, protein and fats – simple really. And, for those times you do eat the packaged, processed 'stuff' – READ THE LABEL!

When to Eat

What's the one thing you can do to get yourself fully alert at all times...energized while remaining calm and relaxed inside? It's eating the right foods AT THE RIGHT TIME. Just as important as what you eat is when you eat it. Timing your meals enhances your energy and focus. Plus it keeps you balanced and able to cope with whatever life is going to throw at you. It really does mean the difference between success and failure.

I get that with your 'on-the-go' schedule it is not easy to keep to certain mealtimes. But eating regularly will help to keep your blood sugar balanced, which keeps you going. Here are a few symptoms of low blood sugar:

- Loss of concentration
- Feeling light headed or dizzy
- Palpitations like your heart is going to burst
- Sweating and feeling extremely weak

Doesn't sound like much fun, does it? Ever felt any of these symptoms before? Well, just a quick little snack (healthy of course) can prevent these symptoms and keep you rocking and rolling. And, please keep in mind these same reactions can sometimes be due to lack of water. Remember your "EIGHTS" from *Chapter Two* and make sure you are drinking enough!

Seriously, most people don't drink enough water, so let me share a bit more information on good old H^2O. It is almost impossible to drink too much water, but your kidneys can only deal with so much at one time...so spread your water consumption throughout the day. You'll know your body has adequate hydration if your urine is clear. That's right, anything colored, dark or smelly means dehydration and possible bacterial infection.

Now, when you start to drink lots of water after a long period of dehydration it may seem like you're peeing a lot. But, once the body has started to absorb the water then this will slow down to a normal pace. Also, realize that some people have a weaker water system than others so don't compare how much you can drink to someone else. Pay attention to your own body.

Check your skin. If it's dry on the outside, chances are you dry on the inside...so drink up. Remember this...tea, coffee and soda are all dehydrating to the body, so the more you drink of that stuff the more water you need to compensate. Okay, enough about drinking...let's take a look at when you should be *eating*.

Back to food: I know you've heard things like "Eat three square meals a day" or "Eat 4 or 5 small meals throughout the day," and maybe even "Just snack throughout the day...whenever you're hungry eat a little something." Okay, is it just me or are those three different ideas of when to eat? Well, let's clear the air and get you the facts. There is one saying, which I know you've heard that is TRUE, TRUE, TRUE!

Breakfast really IS the most important meal of the day - You wouldn't get very far if you didn't put gas in your car, right? So, why think you can run your body on empty? That's just what your body is in the morning...empty. So, this is a must! Do not step out the door to go to school, to practice, to play or even to hang out with your friends if you don't have the correct fuel inside.

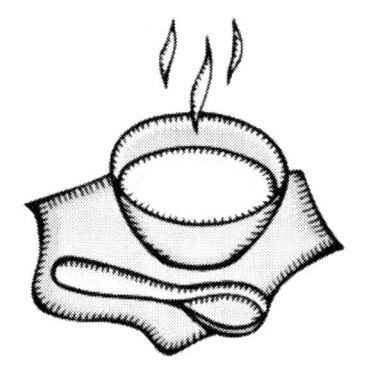

, like oats or muesli and fruit would be perfect (see to make you own really delicious breakfasts). It'll give energy and what you need to sustain your bodily functions and keep your brain active. Lunch and dinner are also important meals and should, of course, be nutritionally sound - based on the list of foods I suggested earlier and your activity for the day. You can check out more about amounts and serving sizes in *How Much to Eat*, the next section of this chapter.

That being said, if you're eating the right portions and starting out with a good breakfast... your 'three squares' is really not the best for keeping your body going and your metabolism humming, unless of course you are slouched in front of the TV or computer.

Imagine your body is a bit like a furnace. Once you've got it burning, you need to keep it burning to stay warm. Waiting too long between meals is like letting the fire in the furnace die down to embers. Then you have to stoke the flames to get things burning again. That's just not very efficient or effective. So...here it is: **The optimum number of meals is really about five...three nutritionally packed meals and two smaller healthy snacks**. It's guaranteed to keep you focused, on fire and ready to take on each step toward your *Healthy Idol* dream!

Healthy Idol

How Much to Eat

Portion Distortion is a real problem! And, it's not really your fault. These days almost everywhere you eat out – especially in America – the portions you're served are WAY out of control. People wanted more for their money, so they got it. The trouble is you don't need it. But, you get used to eating that much food and it becomes 'normal'. It's no wonder so many people – especially young people – have weight issues. Even if you're eating a somewhat decent diet, you're probably eating TOO MUCH!

Here's a quick tip to keep restaurant eating under control:

> The next time you order a meal...ask your server to immediately box half of it for you to take home! That way, even if you eat everything on your plate, it's only half of what they would have served you. That means you've saved calories. Admit it, even if you've told yourself "I won't eat all of this" when food tastes good, it's hard to put the fork down.
>
> So, make the decision before you even see your meal and you'll be a happier, healthier person. Plus, you'll have great leftovers for another meal. Now, with that in mind, let's go over serving sizes and what that really means.

... an average day

- Say breakfast is a cup of muesli (based on my recipe) with a couple of pieces of fruit and a couple of tablespoons of organic natural soy yogurt. That would be an excellent way to start the day. How big a cup? Well just a normal one. I don't really like to get into weighing stuff because how can you take your scales out to the local restaurant! So, start to "weigh things" in your head and begin to visualize correct portions.
- Mid-morning and mid afternoon, maybe a snack of nuts and seeds. They are all different sizes, but about a handful, just the palm of the hand and not heaped up. That's about 4-5 Brazil nuts or 10-15 almonds...you get the idea? Add in some fresh fruit here too – munch on an apple or pear or get some berries in season, maybe raw vegetable sticks and a tub of hummus to dip them into.
- Lunch could be 2-3 cups of vegetable soup (I've included a recipe in **Fact File** C). Nobody gets fat on vegetable soup! You could also try a cup of cooked rice or lentils with a couple of tablespoons of beans, some vegetables and a full salad with a great fresh dressing. Or go for the tortilla wrap full of salad or roasted vegetables. The problem really starts when you add in cheese, meat, chicken or fish because it's easy to eat

- far too much of this. That not only piles on the calories, but adds too much saturated fat as well.
- Your evening meal could consist of something similar. Make your own spicy potato wedges, create a really stunning salad there are recipes in **Fact File** C.
- Carnivores take note!! Try to limit having meat to no more than one portion per day. And, PLEASE make it organic where possible so that you are not eating chemicals, pesticides and hormones in your meal. Eat less meat if possible and get your protein from a vegetable or grain source. Check out the shopping list (**Fact File** B) for some ideas.
- If your age group means that your Mom does all the shopping and cooking, give her this book and go shopping or help her with the cooking so you all get really healthy and don't eat too much of the bad stuff.

Fuel up for exercise…not down time

Now, typical servings and meal sizes aside…there will be times when you may need to adjust how much you eat and get a few more calories into your body. Before you exercise is one of those times. You either already have or you will get conflicting advice as to how you need to fuel up for exercise.

Here's the truth…exercising without real food in your system means your body may use valuable muscle tissue as fuel. That's counterproductive to the whole idea of exercise…which is to build, tone and strengthen the muscle mass you already have. That doesn't mean you should work out on a full stomach...that's not good either. But a small boost of good-for-you carbohydrates about 45 minutes before you work out is ideal. Depending on the time of day, porridge (oatmeal) or muesli, fruit, rice salad, hummus and vegetable sticks or a salad wrap would be great.

Of course, what type of workout you're doing is the key factor to how much energy you'll need, and thereby how much fuel you'll need. But, if you're training hard in the gym, withstanding grueling practices or games on the field or singing away for hours on end, then you will need to be doubly sure about eating the right food at the right time and in the right amount.

Just as important is if you're going to sit in front of a computer or games console many hours on end, then you will need the same high quality food to keep your body systems energized so they can repair, rebuild and renew. But, you won't need as many calories. Listen to your body...it does an amazing job of telling you what it needs. Pay attention to those hunger pangs, any sign of low blood sugar or being overly full. Adjust to what works for you and gets you the steady energy you need to succeed.

Healthy Idol

Are you eating enough?

While thousands of teens and young people are fighting the battle of bulge, too many are also going to the opposite extreme of not getting enough food. The entertainment industry still sends the message that you can't be too thin...and only the skinny bitches of the world will win.

Everyone, mostly you girls – but the guys too, feel the pressure to stay thin and not gain weight. And that it's okay to go to any lengths necessary to accomplish this. With too many bad examples of super skinny, size zero models and actors falling victim to the same hype – it's no wonder you might be tempted to skip a meal (or more). But under nourishing your body is NOT the path to being a Healthy Idol. In fact, based on what we've said about needing food to stay strong and focused, it can really backfire on you.

Some serious illnesses can develop from not eating enough. So, even though so many kids are in need of eating less, I'd be remiss if I didn't address the still too many people who are affected by eating disorders.

I am the first one to admit that my body isn't perfect. I love my curves. Starving myself? So not my thing."
Tyra Banks

Trisha Stewart

Fast Food: Friend or Foe

We've heard on and off for years that junk food is bad...that fast food isn't even real food. But then all those drive-thru joints change their tune and offer 'healthy options' like salads, fruit, yogurt and milk, right? Well, it's time for the truth – whether you're ready to hear it or not. I'll let you know up front that I do NOT advocate going to fast food restaurants. But, I'm not going to just tell you not to go...I'm going to share with you the reasons why. Ultimately, the choice will be yours, but at least you'll have the facts. And, you'll know how that 'burger and fries' can really derail your journey.

Ready? Here goes!

How would you like to seriously increase your risk of cancer, diabetes and heart disease? Check out these scary statistics:

- *Each day in the UK, 6 teenagers are diagnosed with cancer...that's more than 2,000 new cases every year.*
- *Cancer is the most common cause of non-accidental death in teens and young adults in the UK.*
- *1 in 330 boys and 1 in 420 girls will contract cancer before their 20th birthday.*
- *By the age of 15 you have a 1 in 600 chance of developing cancer. By the age of 24 you will have had a 1 in 285 chance of developing cancer.*

Healthy Idol

- *In the last 30 years the incidence of cancer in the teenage and young adult group has increased by 50% and for the first time ever, the number of teens with cancer now exceeds the number of children with cancer.*
- *Teenagers contract some of the most aggressive cancers that are made worse by their growth spurts. (Extract from TCT 2008 (Teenagers Cancer Trust UK))*

Okay, Trisha, you're thinking...those are startling numbers. But, how do you know that diet is linked to cancer? Well, take a look at some of the many studies being done around the world:

- Cancer Research UK has scientific facts that demonstrate the link to poor diet and cancer. Their EPIC (European Prospective Investigation of Cancer) study of more than 500,000 people in 10 European countries has been going on for about 15 years and positively show that diet is very important in the prevention of cancer.
- Excluding skin cancers, colorectal cancer is the third most common cancer diagnosed in both men and women in the United States. *The "American Cancer Society"* estimates that about 108,070 new cases of colon cancer (53,760 in men and 54,310 in women) and 40,740 new cases of rectal cancer (23,490 in men and 17,250 in women) will be diagnosed in 2008.

- A research study at the Dana-Farber Cancer Institute has found a link between diets heavy in red meats, refined breads and desserts and recurring colon cancer. (Doesn't that sound like your typical burger, fries and shake?)

Diabetes, specifically Type 2 diabetes, is on the rise. It leads to heart disease, loss of eye sight, loss of limbs and on-going daily insulin injections. Doesn't sound like much fun, does it? And "IT" will control YOUR life if you get it. And, please read this...more and more teenagers and even younger children are getting this life altering disease. It used to affect mostly adults in their 60s or older. But "Adult Onset Diabetes" has been renamed to "Type 2 Diabetes" due to the increase of younger and younger people suffering with it.

What happens with Type 2 diabetes is that the insulin you produce can't do its job...which is helping the body's cells use glucose for energy. So, your body becomes insulin resistant. That means glucose builds up in the bloodstream and you get high blood sugar. Plus your pancreas keeps producing insulin to try to keep up with your rising blood sugar levels and that can lead to the risk of cardiovascular disease and other health problems.

So, when you're thinking about grabbing a burger and fries from your favorite fast food joint, remember that a study at

Healthy Idol

the Obesity Program at Children's Hospital in Boston indicates that just two fast food meals a week can make you obese and increase your insulin resistance, which leads to Type 2 diabetes.

Heart Disease...think strokes, high cholesterol, heart attacks and high blood pressure. Okay, okay...I realize these symptoms may not be affecting many people under the age of 50. But, you have to know that what you're doing now will affect how healthy you are at 50. And, it's proven fact that diets high in saturated fat lead to blocked arteries, high blood pressure and heart attacks. Remember what I said earlier about trans fats and how they are hidden in so many foods especially from fast food joints and other processed foods.
Guess what? Fast food meals are full of not much more than saturated fats (oh! and some chemicals and sugar). So, if you want to be successful today AND tomorrow, keep your arteries clean and your heart healthy. It's much easier than trying to undo years of damage. And, if you don't think it's that big of a risk, just ask anyone you know who has high blood pressure how worried they are all the time. Or visit the hospitals and see people who have had strokes and have lost the use of half of their body or the ability to speak because part of the brain has died!

I'm sure you're thinking about now...thanks Trisha...that's all really grim stuff. And, what am I supposed to do about that?

Well, let me assure you that these diseases CAN BE PREVENTED. In other words, you do NOT have to end up with diet related cancer, diabetes or heart disease. But, you do have to take the steps necessary to avoid the risk.

Ready to hear how?

Don't eat 'fast food'! Many fast food outlets all have one thing in common: they add massive amounts of highly toxic, mind altering, body challenging preservatives, chemicals, colorings, salt, sugar (especially the worst offender high fructose corn syrup) and hydrogenated (trans) fats to everything they serve.

All of those chemicals, fats, sugars and 'fake food fillers' play havoc on your body and can result in the horrible diseases described above. Please, don't think you're doing okay if you eat the salads they offer…most of them are washed in chlorine water and the dressings are full of chemicals. Where's the real food?

And, don't even get me started on the hygiene side of things. Bacteria and molds can be everywhere…not only those that grow on foods but those introduced by the people who handle the food from factory to your food tray!! There is so much potential sickness, disease and eventual death that could be attributed to eating large amounts of this garbage.

And, since I'm up here on my soap box talking about fast food, let's take a look at those packaged and frozen 'meals' you get at the supermarket. You stick them in the microwave, nuke them up and eat a box full of preservatives, colorings, salt, sugar and whatever else might be called food. Have you ever felt really thirsty after eating this stuff (hmmm, perhaps a tad too much salt??), then you down a fizzy soft drink full of sodium benzoate and masses of some type of sugar. Okay, I'll stop here. But if you want more information about what's really going into your mouth, check out the **Fact File D** in the back of the book (I would if I were you).

Now, of course, I was not born yesterday...nor do I live in some 'TV-Land' 1950's world of every meal being home-cooked. I know you will go to these places with your friends. But, I just cannot bring myself to agree that you could go there once a week, month or whatever. In fact, I believe those "fast chemical factory" places should be closed down. I know you probably don't agree with me there...at least not yet. So, in the meanwhile I have come up with a solution for those of you with no willpower to stay out!!!

Whew! Okay, I feel a bit better having shared my rant with you...and it's the truth. That's why I had to share it. But, I also have to share my answer for a fast food binge. First, you will be a bit better off if you stick with the salads and such in these places (not ideal, but certainly better). But if you find you've weakened and wolfed down a burger combo or something, take the next day to completely cleanse your system. Please use my

"Healthy Idol Detox". Your poor kidneys, your overworked liver and your struggling immune system will thank you. This is what I recommend you do after eating fast food or drinking bad stuff:

Healthy Idol Detox

- Juice on only organic fruits and vegetables and take 1000mgs of vitamin C for the day.
- Eat some wholegrain rice with beans and lentils.
- Drink around 2 liters of filtered water.

This will balance the ph of the body and bring you back to feeling great again. It may sound over the top but if you consider how many years you are likely to be on this planet then it makes sense to take good care of yourself. Doing a one day 'detox' is also a good way to help your body rest, revamp and revitalize after too much stress, too many long hours or whatever else might get you off-kilter.

Cool Substitutes for Junk Food

Okay, this may not be what you think it's going to be. There aren't really any cool, tasty packaged foods that are real and healthy. However, I believe with a bit of effort, imagination and self control you can make anything you like from real foods. They'll taste great and be cheaper. That's a major plus as fast food is also expensive. So if you are a student sharing a house with other students or you're living at home you can still have healthy foods on hand, regardless of budget.

So, here are a few ideas:

1. Stock up on healthy fast foods like unsalted nuts, dates, fresh coconut, fruit, real maple syrup, carob powder, vanilla extract, fresh ginger, avocado and guess what, you can blend or crush all of these ingredients to make cookies, smoothies, juices and so on. You will probably need some recipes so check out the new Healthy Bunch Cookbook.
2. Expand your idea of fast food...think beyond the burger, taco or chicken shack to include Greek kebabs or pitas, a local sandwich shop that uses local, fresh ingredients, or get a baked potato with fresh toppings
3. Visit a smoothie or juice bar where the fruit/vegetables are whizzed up in front of you - no cheating going on there, just good whole food.
4. Check out the whole food/vegetarian cafe/restaurants in your area. There are more and more out there and most are very

competitively priced. They offer a variety of sandwiches, wraps and salads.
5. Visit the international district in your city (or wherever you can find the authentic cultural cuisines). Most of these small cafes and eateries use real, authentic ingredients without chemicals and preservatives. Just go light on the sauces if you're not sure. And, many offer vegetarian dishes that are tasty options.
6. Find an Asian café that offers Edamame (crunchy, sweet soy beans in the pod) and munch away
7. Make this real fun by checking new places and recommending them to your friends!
8. Supplements – just a quick word on those while we are talking food. Vitamins and mineral supplements can be very expensive to take on a regular basis. And, if you follow the guidelines in this book, you shouldn't need them anyway. However, if you are seriously burning up all your fuel in a demanding situation (like strenuous exercise or intense sports) then it may be advisable to take supplements to be sure you're body is getting all the nutrition it needs.

Of course, there are so many supplements on the market that are absolute rubbish. That's why getting a supply of good quality vitamins and minerals is essential, and will actually save you money in the long run. Don't be fooled by all the ads you see. If you need a good supplement, visit my website (www.trishastewart.com) for the best of what's out there. My team has researched them thoroughly and will give you the truth. Also, don't buy into the idea that the shakes or protein drinks you can buy are suitable supplements that will help you build muscle, lose weight or whatever. There is nothing that will replace a really good diet and exercise program.

Now that you've got the basics for what, when and how much to eat - plus what to avoid (I know you know what I'm talking about) - you can get started on eating your way to being a Healthy Idol. Of course, its more than just food...but fueling yourself the right way is vital to having the strength, endurance and drive to do the rest. So, grab a healthy snack and let's move on to the power of exercise!

Chapter 4

Exercise

There are NO Idle Idols

"I'm very dedicated to staying in shape when I'm on tour. In fact, last year my crew staged an intervention to try to get me to stop going to the gym so much. I just get so into it. I love to sweat and I love to feel like a beast."
Pop Rocker - Pink

So, you think her lyrics "I can go for miles, if you know what I mean," just refers to being on the treadmill? Okay, maybe she's goes to the extreme...I mean, an intervention for working out? But, you can't argue with the results...she looks FABULOUS! And, if you think a life of touring is easy on the body...you're wrong. As far as partying all the time...forgettaboutit!! Not if you expect to last!

Wait...don't throw the book down! I'm not saying you can't ever have a good time and celebrate. But remember your body is your instrument... keep it in playing condition.

It's really quite simple...**Healthy Idols** don't just sit around and wait for things to happen for them...they go out there and get to work. That goes for being fit and strong as well, which is a big part of being a **Healthy Idol**. But fitness doesn't just

Healthy Idol

happen...not even for Halle Berry! Seriously, have you ever seen the extreme workout regime she stuck to while getting in shape for the movie **Catwoman**? Okay, the movie wasn't so great, but you've got to admit...she looked AMAZING! So, we can look to the many role models out there in the "Idol" world to figure out how we should get into shape...right?

SLOW DOWN...it really depends on who you're looking at...so look closely. Some of our greatest icons of the entertainment industry could never be labeled **Healthy Idols**. Unfortunately, most are not known for hitting the gym. They're known for hitting the hot spots, checking into rehab, doing jail time for DUIs or, sadly, dying from drug overdoses. Way too many talented people are making poor choices that shorten and (too often) end their careers. Those stars may burn brightly, but they burn too quickly and are then gone. That's not what I want for you at all. I want you to have the complete package...what it takes to be successful and remain healthy for the long haul!

And, trust me – there are some celebrities out there who are doing it right! Women like Jennifer Garner, Sheryl Crow, Madonna and our favorite feline – Halle Berry are strong and sexy. Male celebrities who keep 'lean and mean' include Will Smith, Usher, Daniel Craig (the new James Bond) and Matt Damon. So, ask yourself two questions:

1. Do you want to be a Healthy Idol that has the staying power for decades of success?
2. Do you want to avoid the lifestyle pitfalls that lead us to weight issues and obesity, diabetes, heart attacks and even untimely death?

Yes?! Good. Then do this...GET UP OFF THE COUCH AND GET MOVING!! I'm serious, put down the remote, the joystick, the controller, the computer mouse, your iPod or cell phone. Whatever it is that keeps you stuck on the sofa...turn it off.

It's okay, it will still be there when you get back. Please, stop playing video games and just go play! Stop texting and start walking. Get off MySpace and get outside. To be the best you can be you need to exercise! It not only makes you look good, but you'll feel good as well (that's the beauty of endorphins or happy hormones).

The Benefits of Movin' It

Your body was meant to move! Don't ignore that. Most of you reading this book are still maturing and developing, both physically and mentally. Helping your bones, brain and muscle to grow strong is a smart move. And, if you don't start exercising now...opting for that couch potato, computer zombie, video coma lifestyle...you won't like the results. Chances are that with all that 'down time' you'll end up being shorter, have back problems and body fat problems. Now, I've

Healthy Idol

already said it will make you feel better...but let me give you some more general benefits:

- Tones and builds muscles
- Makes you stronger
- Improves circulation
- Speeds up metabolism
- Burns fat
- Strengthen bones
- Improves self-esteem (more confidence)
- Relieves stress
- Provides on-going energy
- Regulates hormones
- Helps mood highs and lows
- Keeps you clean (great deterrent to stay off drugs & alcohol)
- Enhances your physical and mental growth

Here are some specific benefits for girls and guys!
Okay, ladies...it's REALLY important you exercise because you constantly have to deal with the ups and downs of becoming a woman. And, with the extreme amount of pressure to be stick thin, you need all the support and tools to keep focused on a positive healthy image...and that's what a good workout is all about.

Trisha Stewart

Remember that exercising and working out doesn't mean you'll end up looking like a guy. I'll give you some things to do that will help you become strong and empowered!

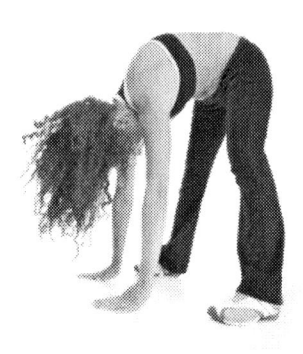

> *"Being a size 0 doesn't make you beautiful.*
> *To all girls with butts, boobs, hips and a waist, put on a bikini -*
> *put it on and stay strong."*
> **Jennifer Love Hewitt**, *star of 'The Ghost Whisperer'*

Now for the guys! I know some of you may actually want to pump yourself up and get ripped muscles and there's nothing wrong with that as long as you do it the right way (more on that in a bit). But, even if that's not the look for you...you can be strong, lean and healthy. Working out will give your muscles great shape, boosts your confidence and let's be honest...make you more attractive. And, keep in mind that as you reach maturity your raging hormones will also benefit from regular exercise.

Healthy Idol

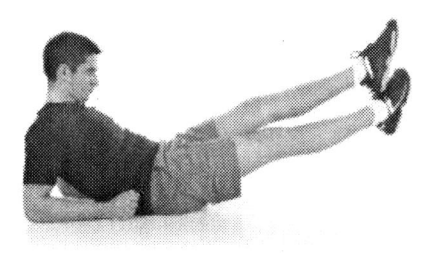

So benefits aside, that doesn't mean you have to take hours of aerobics classes or hit the gym to lift as much weight as you possibly can. I've got some great ideas for getting started and making it easy, fun and affordable...just read on. Plus, I've worked with the Trisha Stewart Team Personal Trainer, Christin McDowell, and we've put together some great information on the website (www.TrishaStewart.com) including workouts, tips and answers to your toughest questions. So, ready to get started?

Gym or No Gym...ways to get going

There are lots of ways to get your heart pumping and get some exercise into your daily life. You can join a gym, play sports, dance...but let's start with some even more basic ideas. If you're not used to exercise, the thought of organized sports or taking a class may be a bit intimidating. I get that. So take a look at these ideas:

Trisha Stewart

Ten Steps to add fitness to everyday activities

1. Walk to where you're going! Be safe...don't go alone and don't go further than you should for your age. Check with your parents to get the okay before you ever head out the door!!).
2. Skip the elevator and take the stairs (eventually run up or take them two at a time)
3. Whether you're driving or someone else...park further away from the entrance to get in a few extra steps.
4. Take your dog (or the neighbor's dog) for a walk. Even 20 minutes will help you and Fido feel better.
5. Walk around your block and time yourself...try to do it faster each time.
6. PLAY...hit the playground and have some fun on the monkey bars (if you feel a bit old for that...do it on a weekend when no one's around!)
7. Dance! Turn on your favorite tunes and move around the room. Don't worry if you don't know the latest steps...close the door and groove in by yourself in your bedroom.
8. Mow the yard/lawn and rake the clippings. Or if it's fall/autumn...rake the leaves! Yard work is a great workout and you'll win big points for keeping the yard looking good. And while we're at it, how about washing your car? Why pay at the car wash

when it's a great workout. You'll look good and your car will look great too.
9. Vacuum. If it's too cold or rainy to mow, you can clean the carpets and get a good cardio workout!
10. Pull the bicycle out of the garage and take it for a spin!

The Basics of Getting Started
Whether you're working to become an award-winning singer or a pro-athlete...you need to have a plan for your training. So, keep a few things in mind: Have a goal, create a program, be focused, stay positive, be smart and HAVE FUN.

And please NO: workouts over 2 hours, sports drinks (they're all sugar or fake sugar), steroids, diet pills or protein bars (eat real food)!

AND READ THIS: You DON'T have to go to the gym to have a great workout. There are tons of things you can do without ever stepping foot into a gym. What are the things you like to do or have always wanted to try? Here are some of those ideas:
- Skateboarding, snowboarding, wake boarding-anything to do with a board
- Rollerblading or ice skating
- Soccer, basketball, racquetball, volleyball, softball, tennis, football...any type of sport

- Hiking or rock climbing
- Walking, running, sprinting
- Swimming, scuba diving, diving
- Biking: road, mountain, BMX or dirt biking
- Yoga, Pilates, Tai Chi, martial arts, kick boxing and more

Do what you love...or try something new. I would recommend doing any of these activities as many times a week as possible.

Weighing in on weight training

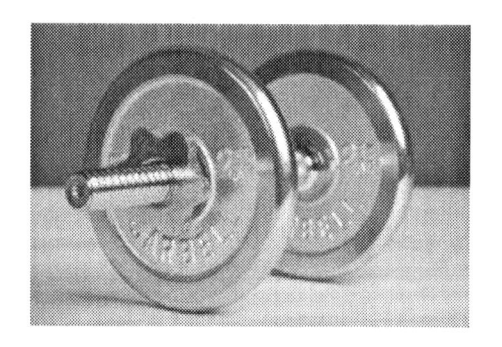

I know some of you are going to want to lift some weights. If you're interested, please visit the website (www.TrishaStewart.com) for more specific guidance and support. However, keep in mind that I do not recommend heavy weight training for anyone under the age of 16. You do not want to restrict normal development of certain muscles. Plus there are plenty of 'body weight' exercises that build muscle, like pushups and squats (again, there's more information on the website).

Healthy Idol

Get fit fast!

Okay, if you're ready to make a real difference to your body...two of the quickest ways to get in shape are running and swimming! If you are not a "runner"...don't worry you can become one. And you don't have to be a long distance runner or sprinter to run. You can do whatever you want! Here are some good running ideas:

- Run with a friend you know will be consistent, hold you accountable and challenge you.
- Run on a track or dirt rather than pavement (it's easier on your body).
- Get the right running shoes....shoes that offer good support and are lightweight. If you have access to someone who can do a running gait analysis on you, do it! To prevent or reduce the possibility of shin splints and other kinds of strain, inserts are often a good idea for your running shoes. The company 'Foot Zone' can tell you what kind of inserts you should wear inside your shoes. Otherwise, just go to a reputable store for help. Remember to get new running shoes every six months or so if you can afford them. It's a worthwhile investment.
- If you are new to running or maybe even hate it. Give it a shot. When you're out for a walk, try to run for a certain amount of time, say 20 seconds. Walk again and then run

for 20 more seconds. Eventually increase the time you're running.

If you love to run, then here's a sample fitness running program. If you can't do it at this time, build up to it.

- Run 400m (one lap around a typical track)
- Walk 100m (one straight or one curved segment of the track
- Repeat 3 times
    - Run Fast 200m (half lap)
    - Walk 100m (quarter lap)
    - Repeat 2 times
        - Run Very Fast 100m
        - Walk 25m
        - Repeat 5 times
            - Run 400-800m (one to two laps)
            - Repeat 1-2 times

Swimming is a wonderful tool to help lean out, lengthen and "tone" your body. If you don't know how to swim, get a coach, join a swim class at school or get pointers from a lifeguard. Check with your high school, if you have a pool, to see when you can use it. Also, most communities have a neighborhood pool. If you have a friend who knows how to swim, ask him or her to go with you and make it a time to get some great

Healthy Idol

activity but also spend time together. I promise you, swimming will make you feel wonderful!

Here's a sample swim program:

Note:

> - 1 lap is 50 m, down and back
> - 25m is just down, unless you are using a full sized Olympian pool; which are rare!

- Swim 100m
- Jog in the deep end 30 Sec.
- Rest then repeat 3-4 times
  - Swim fast 25m-50m
  - Recover then Repeat 5 times
    - Swim 100m
    - Repeat 1-4 times
      - Kick 50m

And please - no matter your goal or vision of how buff you'll be - do NOT worry if your legs are not as long as your favorite model or football idol, or you seem to carry more weight on the legs than your friend or perhaps your buddy has a larger chest expansion than you.

These are all genetics, which means it's the way you were born. Remember, if everyone looked the same it would be incredibly boring. What you can do is make yourself the best for your body shape and type and you WILL look incredible.

And, don't forget, you may be still growing. So, just get started and have lots of fun. Stick with things you enjoy so you'll be more inclined to keep it up. And, add some variety to keep it interesting...inside, outside, team sports, solo workouts...just keep moving.

If you really want to get into great shape, then checkout Christin McDowell's workout book, 'Healthy Fitness Central'.

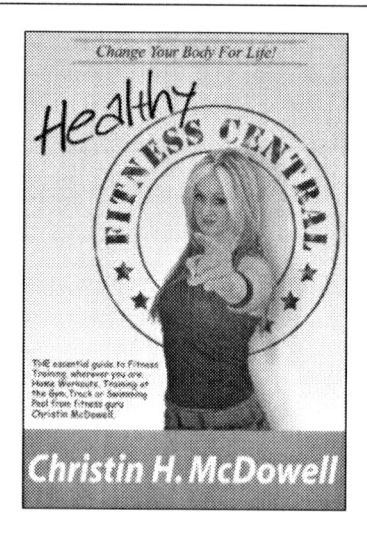

Chapter 5

Everything Else

> *"Drugs have nothing to do with the creation of music. In fact, drugs are dumb and self-indulgent.*
> *Kind of like sucking your thumb."*
> **Courtney Love**

Sex, Drugs & Rock n' Roll

Well, I guess that sort of sums it up...doesn't it? Substances like alcohol and drugs are really just things people use to try to feel better...or feel nothing at all. They do not...let me repeat that - NOT...make you more talented, smarter, cooler, prettier or better in anyway. But, despite that, everyone seems to be trying something and overdoing it. So, as Courtney Love might say, let's take the thumbs out of our mouths and get real about 'everything else' that you have to deal with on your way to becoming a Healthy Idol!

Okay, I'd have my head literally stuck in the ground like an ostrich (avoiding the obvious) if I didn't think you were dealing with some very real pressures about sex, drugs and drinking. These days it seems that decisions about these life changing practices are being made by younger and younger kids. But, don't worry...I'm not going to go on about how drugs are illegal as is underage drinking...you already know that.

What I am going to share with you is the truth about drugs, sexually transmitted diseases and alcohol. I want you to know the truth about what these things can do to your body, your mind and, most sadly...your future. Here's the thing...you're on your way to being a Healthy Idol and I want to see you make it to the top. You've got a vision, a dream, some great goals and developing talent. Don't get derailed by making poor choices. If you don't think it can happen to you, it can. Do you really think that Lindsey Lohan planned to end up a repeat rehab customer? What about Amy Winehouse? Do you realize she had to get special permission to get out of her treatment center so she could perform at the Grammys? Talk about having to put your life and dreams on hold! And, let's not forget about those lives that have been cut short...those great talents we'll never see ripen to old age including Chris Farley, River Phoenix and Heath Ledger.

That's why I want to share the truth about what can happen to you. With that you can make better informed decisions. And, I'm going to offer a few places for you to turn if you're having problems. So, even if you've made a few bad choices along the way...it's not too late. Let's get you back on track and on your way to being the best you!

SEX

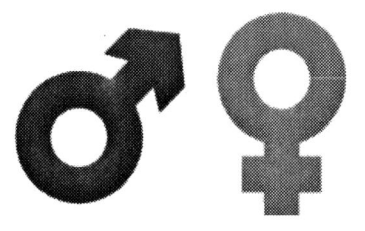

Now that I have your attention, let me say that I'm not going to try to convince you when you should or shouldn't have sex. There are certainly ages that are too young to shoulder the responsibility and the emotional weight sex carries with it (that means it's more than just the physical act, it's how you feel about yourself and the other person afterwards). Those decisions are personal and I hope you have a parent or trusted adult you can talk to if you're thinking about having sex for the first time. Do remember this though...

DON'T LET ANYONE PRESSURE YOU TO DO SOMETHING YOU ARE NOT READY TO DO!

I don't care if you're male or female, if you don't feel ready...take a moment, say no and then walk away. Anyone who truly cares about you will respect your decision. Okay, there I've said it. Now, let me bust one myth that still floats around out there.

There's a rumor that keeps popping up that you can't get pregnant the first time you have sex, or that you can't catch an

STD (sexually transmitted disease) the first time. WRONG!! Anything that can happen as a result of having sex can happen the first time you have it. So, with that in mind, let's take a look at some of the things that can happen to you when you have sex:

First, of course is the obvious result of getting pregnant...and I hope I don't need to tell you that becoming a parent while you're still growing up yourself is beyond difficult. And, boys, don't think this is only a worry for the young girls out there. It takes two to make a baby and it takes two to handle the responsibility of what happens after that.

Even if you don't get pregnant, there are a host of life altering diseases you can get...and there's no gender (or even age) preference here. STDs affect as many women as men from all age groups! And, STDs can spread through any type of sexual activity involving the sex organs or the mouth. In fact, infection can also be spread through contact with blood during sexual activity. So, there really is no such thing as safe sex. But, are STDs really a concern for you? Well think about this:

- Kids are becoming sexually active at much younger ages and are having sex with a greater number of partners.
- You can be symptom free and STILL pass STDs to sexual partners.
- STDs in women can lead to infertility and an increased chance of cervical cancer.

Healthy Idol

- It is possible, especially if having lots of partners, that you can attract more than one type of STD - that means a major whammy on your health and immunity.

Okay, what are some of the most common STDs that can impact your life? Well, for those of you who LOVE details, I've put together some information in **Fact File** F (see the back of the book) with lots of facts and data for you to review. However, for those you who roll their eyes at the thought of lots of numbers and statistics, I've just put the highlights in this chapter.

Gonorrhea It's one of the most common diseases passed from one person to another during sexual activity. There are not always symptoms, especially for women, but painful urination is a big warning sign. More than 5% of people between 18 and 35 have gonorrhea and DON'T EVEN KNOW IT. The scary thing is that it can spread to other parts of the body and cause real complications, and new strains are resisting treatment even with strong antibiotics!

Chlamydia THE most common STD in the United States, about 5% of the ENTIRE population is infected and about 10% sexually active teenage girls! And, guess who those girls are having sex with...teenage boys...so it affects the guys too! It can lead to chronic pelvic pain and even infertility if not treated.

Genital Herpes Herpes is a highly infectious disease that causes blisters or small sores on and around the genitals...not fun at all. It cannot be cured, only controlled. And, you can spread herpes even if you are not suffering from an active breakout...that's why there are as many as one million new infections.

HIV/AIDS Probably the scariest of all STDs...there is no cure for HIV, which can lead to AIDS. This disease attacks your immune system and weakens your ability to fight off even the simplest infections. So any infection or illness can become life threatening. HIV can be spread through sexual intercourse, blood transfusions or sharing drug needles with an infected person.

Hepatitis Hepatitis (A B and C) is a general term that means inflammation of the liver. The most common strain transmitted sexually (through semen or saliva) is Hepatitis B. Again, people may show no signs of illness, but can still spread the disease. While it can be treated, the younger you are when you contract it, the more likely you will face

Healthy Idol

chronic (or on-going) Hepatitis B and that can lead to a host of other illnesses. Check out **Fact File** F for more details on all three types of Hepatitis.

So, here's the deal...you WILL contract one or more of these STD's if:

- you are sharing needles to take illegal drugs,
- having multiple sex partners and not using condoms,
- men having sex with men and not using condoms,
- women having sex with an infected person,
- drinking contaminated water or
- Eating food that has been handled by someone contaminated with the virus.

Clearly, the ideal way to eliminate the risk of getting an STD is to abstain for sex. But, like I said before, that's a decision you have to make for yourself. But be smart; think it through completely before you make a decision. And, if you're not yet convinced of the dangers...check out **Fact File** D.

DRUGS

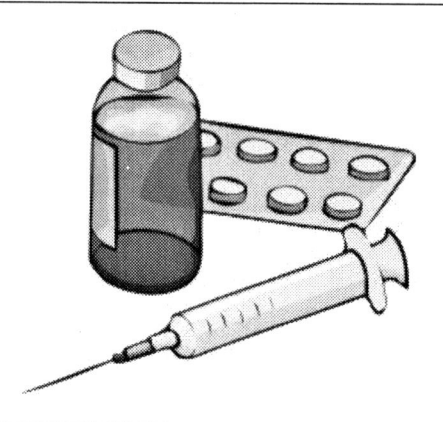

> "I would never do crack... I would never do a drug named after a part of my own ass, okay?"
> **Denis Leary**

More young people are using drugs than ever before...and these drugs are more than the illegal substances bought on a shady street corner. Sure marijuana is still out there, but drug abuse has expanded to include inhalants, steroids and even prescription drugs that are intended to help people.

Seriously, the number of teens abusing prescription drugs more than tripled from 1992 to 2003. That number climbs daily and does not include teenagers using illegal drugs, the whole situation is frightening. I want to be sure you know the impact drugs...all drugs...can have on your life and how they can bring your Healthy Idol dreams to an end.

Healthy Idol

Now, if I tried to talk about every substance that can be abused...well, that would be a book all by itself. So, instead I'm just going to highlight some of the most common drugs and their ill effects (and I've included some great resources and statistics in **Fact File** E).

Marijuana Lots of people think marijuana or 'pot' is harmless. I mean come on; they even use it for medical pain relief in cancer patients, right? Well, before you make your final decision, let me share a few of the effects smoking a joint or two:

- Impaired short-term memory
- Impaired attention, judgment, and other cognitive functions
- Impaired coordination and balance
- Increased heart rate
- Impaired memory and learning skills
- Hallucinations if taking massive doses
- Possible addiction
- Increased risk of chronic cough, bronchitis, and emphysema
- Increased risk of cancer of the head, neck, and lungs

Inhalants From hair spray and spray paint to correction fluid and felt tip pens...nearly 10% of teens ages 12 – 17 have abused inhalants. Effects include confusion...nosebleeds...headaches ...loss of hearing and sense of smell...severe mood swings...violent behavior...and the worst side effect - death **(READ THIS...55% of deaths were first time users!)**

Hallucinogens There are many different kinds of hallucinogens. Some occur naturally, in trees, vines, seeds, fungi and leaves...others are manufactured in laboratories. But, there is one thing they all have in common - they are very dangerous. Here's a list and some of their slang names:

- LSD (lysergic acid diethylamide) - Acid, trips, microdots, dots.
- Magic mushrooms (psilocybin) - golden tops, blue meanies, liberty caps
- Morning glory seeds
- Mescaline (peyote cactus)
- PCP (phencyclidine) - Angel dust, peace pill.
- Ketamine - Special K, K, ket, kitkat, super K
- Ecstasy (MDMA and related drugs, in high doses)
- Cannabis – marijuana (in high quantities)

So, what are some of the effects of using hallucinogens? Try these on for size: violent sickness and diarrhea, panic attacks, confusion, mental disturbances, heart attack, epileptic fits and more...none of which sounds much fun.

Stimulants Most stimulants are prescribed by a doctor and intended to help those who take them...from kids with ADHD (Attention Deficit Hyperactive Disorder) to people battling obesity. But, these stimulants – like too many prescription drugs – are being misused and abused by people who shouldn't be taking them in the first place. And, of course there are illegal stimulants like methamphetamines, cocaine/crack and crystal meth that are extremely powerful. And, because they are easily tolerated and very addictive...once you start taking them you need more and more. And, the resulting effects can be extreme and permanent from restlessness to paranoia to psychosis.

Depressants Like stimulants...some depressants are prescribed to treat certain problems. Sedatives and barbiturates address sleeplessness, anxiety, tension and help prevent epileptic seizures. Of course, these can easily be abused and often are due to their highly addictive nature. Long term dependence causes impaired memory and judgment, hostility, depression, mood swings, chronic fatigue, and the stimulation of pre-existing emotional disorders, which may result in paranoia or thoughts of suicide.

Steroids Here's the thing...taking steroids is just NOT a smart thing to do. Why do you think they're making such a big deal about it in major league sports? Your body naturally makes steroids and that's all you need for growth and development. Adding to that by taking anabolic steroids can cause some majorly negative side effects. Don't believe me? Along with developing high blood pressure, jaundice and liver tumors, here are some gender specific symptoms to think about:

- Men - Shrinking testicles, reduced sperm count, infertility, baldness, development of breast tissue and an increased risk of prostate cancer.
- Women – facial hair, male pattern baldness, menstrual cycle issues, enlarged clitoris and a deepened voice.
- And teens that take steroids risk altered or halted growth...that means you can end up shorter than you should. No wonder it's such a scary statistic that nearly 30% of 8th – 12th graders are using anabolic steroids.

Healthy Idol

There are also other types of steroids that you could be using and not even know it. From bronchial inhalers and nasal sprays to creams, pills and shots, steroid therapy is used to treat a variety of illnesses, but the side effects can be horrifying and permanent. Check out **Fact File** G for a complete listing of steroid use symptoms.

Smoking/Nicotine Smoking is the primary cause of cancer, everyone knows that but did you know it is as addictive as any other drug? That's why it's the most difficult habit to kick...so the best bet is to never start. Plus, you can lose some of your ability to taste and smell and have some serious digestive problems.

Caffeine Okay, so this one isn't illegal...but it's a true stimulant and can be quite addictive. It's in coffee, tea, sodas, some pain killers and diet aids. What does it do? Caffeine raises blood pressure, can give you the shakes, headaches, sleep disorders and can cause anxiety attacks.

Whew - I know that's a lot of information...but there's still more. Again, for those who want the details and more facts...take a peek at **Fact File** E...especially if you're still thinking a little drug use is okay.

Skin Deep...Taking Care of the Outside Package

Healthy Idols focus on being healthy on the inside, but I'd be lying if I said how you look on the outside isn't a part of your entire ***Healthy Idol*** package. Of course others have opinions on your looks, but what really matters is how you feel about yourself. And that feeling can hit rock bottom if your skin, hair and nails aren't at their best. But here's the truth...what goes on the inside dictates what happens on the outside.

So following the right eating plan (remember Chapter 3?) will cause your skin to be clear, eyes bright, nails strong and hair flowing. Plus, another major benefit, you won't have smelly feet or armpits! Now there are tons of products on the market that promise the best looking skin and hair ever, but I promise you there is only one solution you need. And, that's the one you have already been reading about in this book...the Four Foundation Stones...eating right, exercising, plenty of rest and water!

Now, for any of you just starting on your journey I've provided some helpful tips and information...because wherever you're starting point is...you just need to get started.

Face and Body

- If you have pimples, bumps or clogged pores, don't squeeze them. It may cause scarring and open wounds which could lead to infection making the problem twice as bad.
- Do not use the strong chemical cleansers that can dry your skin and cause peeling and make an unsightly mess.
- Scrubbing with a light natural abrasive cream like almond or a fine salt scrub will help to remove dead skin, allow the skin to breathe and eliminate any natural wastes far more efficiently.
- Keep your face clothes or sponges clean at all times, this will prevent any bacteria forming and being transferred to your skin.
- Remember your Eights…getting enough sleep, rejuvenates your skin
- Use only natural cleansers without added chemicals (hit the Internet and search for natural products).
- Get a massage every now and again, this will not only feel wonderful but will help with circulation and relaxation.

Feet

- Keep your nails and cuticles trimmed and clean.
- Give your feet a good scrub with a natural salt scrub at least once a week.
- Use a pumice or other abrasive product to get rid of any hard skin as this will prevent good circulation to those areas.
- Get a foot massage and or a pedicure...your feet will look good and feel great!
- Exercise those feet; keep the joints open and the muscles stretched.
- Don't wear shoes that don't fit right. And, if you wear high heels a lot make sure spend some time barefoot to stretch the Achilles tendon and your toes.

Hands and Nails

- Keep your fingernails clean...it looks better and ensures you're not carrying around hidden bacteria. Bacteria that's unhealthy for you AND others if you make them something to eat...think about it...eeewww!
- Have a manicure once a week...whether you do it yourself or hire a professional. Its how you can keep your cuticles nicely shaped and trimmed; and file any ragged or unsightly edges off your nails.

Healthy Idol

- Use a mild abrasive and give them a good scrub once a week, this will get rid of dead skin and make them look fabulous!
- Eating right makes your nails grow faster...so keep up with your trims.
- Put moisture cream or lotion on several times daily...especially if you're outside or have to wash your hands a lot.
- Exercise your hands and stretch them out to keep the joints open and the muscles flexible.

Hair

- Do not use strong shampoos (for dandruff, oily hair, etc.) as they're too hard on your hair and completely unnecessary. Use a natural shampoo and conditioner with no chemicals added, and you can check out the Internet to find some great natural products.
- Wash hair regularly, but not too much. Once every couple of days is enough. And, if you feel your hair is excessively oily...it could be related to your diet – so look closely at what you're eating.
- Invest in getting a great stylist to cut your hair...it's worth it to have someone who really knows what they're doing help you create the right look for you!
- Cover your hair in extreme sunlight because otherwise it will dry out (or fade any color you've had done).

And, if you'll be out for a while...put some good moisture treatment on your hair while it's covered...it'll be in even better condition.

- Wear a cap if you swim a lot...great for the body...but the chlorine is too hard on your hair. It can actually CHANGE color...especially if your hair has been color treated. Do you want greenish-blonde hair...seriously?

Oral

Bad breath is definitely not "cool," but most people think it's in their mouth...so chew gum or eat mints to 'fix it." For some, the problem may actually be deeper in the digestive system, but for now let's get focused on the mouth (teeth, gums and tongue). Because, you have been reading this book and that means you know the 'healthy and good' foods to eat.

Brush and floss your teeth twice a day! How many times do you remember being told that one? From your parents, your dentist, even most toothpaste products tell you right on the package. So, what's so important about brushing and flossing? Sure it can help our teeth be brighter and whiter...but let's think about what happens if you don't.

Have you ever really looked at your teeth? They have nooks and crannies and crevices where bacteria can hide and build up. Did you know that 'oral bacteria' is linked to heart disease, diabetes and blood infections? So, brushing your teeth is about

Healthy Idol

more than a bright smile and fighting bad breath...which by the way can definitely be a sign that something else is going awry with your body. Bacteria can lead to gum disease...and then all that bacteria and those toxins can get into your blood system.

You can end up with a low grade infection, inflammation, pain and more. That's an attack on your body that can weaken your immune system...opening the door to ill health. Bottom line...when your dentist says brush and floss...do it!!

Maintaining your 'outer package' doesn't have to be complicated, just consistent. So, when you follow the ideas I've described here and use natural products as much as possible, you're going to look and feel great.

Sure, there will be times when you don't feel your best...pressure from school, friends and just working hard for your big break can wear you down. At those times, you may find yourself making some not so smart choices about how you care for your body. Don't beat yourself up...just get back on track and start again. Keep coming back to the basics, re-read this book and visit the website (www.trishastewart.com)...the answers and support you'll need are there.

Chapter 6

OBSTACLES

> "These parents, they think I'm a role model for their kids...that their kids look at me as some sort of idol. But it's the parents' job to make sure their kids don't turn out that shallow. That's not my responsibility. I'm not responsible for your kid."
> **Britney Spears**

Whew! Well, no matter your thoughts about Britney she makes a valid point, doesn't she? So, if Britney isn't watching out for you, who is? Guess what? Even with all the right support and a team of family and friends to back you...it comes down to one person. YOU! Great...one more thing for your 'to do' list: right? But think about it...you're the one who has to make the decisions...even when you have help sorting through all your options (which by the way...you should. Don't skip the section in Chapter 7 about NOT going it alone!). But read this first!

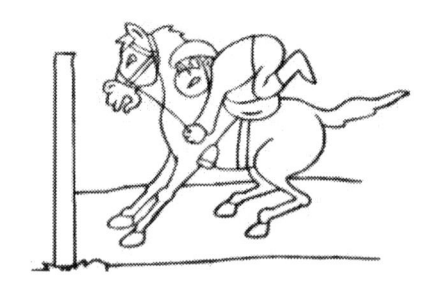

Healthy Idol

When you really want something, it's worth working for...and it's often a lot of work that comes with setbacks, struggles and obstacles. So before you think that all you have to do is set your sights, make your plans and move ahead...slow down. Realize that some days will be really hard, some days you'll feel like no one is on your side and sometimes you might just want to give up. DON'T! Since we know those bumps in the road are coming up...let's look at what they are so you'll be better prepared to deal with them.

Peer Pressure

Everyone deals with peer pressure...to be honest most us have a bit of time on both the giving and receiving end. And, I know there is sometimes positive peer pressure...like friends who encourage you to study for your final exam. But, as we're talking about obstacles here, let's take a look at negative peer pressure.

Where does peer pressure come from? The idea is that it is your 'peers,' people on your level and that means your friends and siblings. But in reality, peer pressure is a bit broader than that because pressure comes from people all around you and it often gets filtered down through your friends.

You may have already dealt with your share of peer pressure, but don't think that it's over. There are always people out there ready and willing to lead you down the wrong path and encourage you to choose the fast, easy and sometimes wrong option. Here are just a few scenarios you're likely to face as you strive to achieve your **Healthy Idol** status and some tips on how to deal with them:

- Everyone's going out to the fast food joint for burgers and they insist to you that one combo meal isn't going to hurt you. *After reading my information on fast food, hopefully you do know that this junk food should never cross your lips...so stay strong by picking a more healthy café, bringing your own snacks or...worst case scenario...committing to the 24-hour 'post fast food' cleanse/detox in Chapter 3.*
- You've got practice or rehearsal after school, but your friends want you to hang out with them instead. They tell you that if you're really their friend, you'd want to spend time with them. *This is hard, because sometimes your friends get jealous when you achieve things and do well. They unknowingly sabotage your success by trying to lead you astray.*

  Assure your friends you do care about them and make specific plans together for another time. If they persist, remind them that if they were YOUR friends, they'd understand how important your goals are and encourage you to keep at it.
- You get pressured about having sex before you're ready. This can happen from the person you're

Healthy Idol

dating...that's the obvious pressure. But, these days you can get pressure from your friends as they insist 'everyone's doing it' and you should just 'go for it.'

The pressure to have sex can be overwhelming...especially when you have strong, romantic feelings for someone. This is when you do NOT need to go it alone! Find someone to talk to (check out more ideas on getting support in Chapter 7)! This is a major decision that can have life changing consequences... so be sure you really know what's right for you.

o This one is especially, but not exclusively, for young women. You and your friends all want to be thinner because you're hoping to look like some celebrity or super model. Someone suggests using diet pills, laxatives, bulimia (throwing up what you eat) or encourages not eating at all.

There's nothing wrong with having goals to be fitter, leaner and healthier...as long as you keep it in perspective. Remember that you'll need strength and stamina to sing, dance, and play sports, whatever. Food is the fuel to give you that strength. Find fitness magazines that show strong models for you and your friends to admire. And, remind yourself that you want to be around for a long time...fad diets, pills and being too thin will shorten your life.

- There's a new video or computer game out and everyone's playing it. Your friends want to sit around playing it for HOURS and they want you right there with them...doing nothing but sitting on the couch and eating snacks. *If you love games and like your friends...there's nothing wrong with spending time with both. However, remember 'all things in moderation'.*

  Sitting too long undoes all the good you've done with eating right and exercising, so set a time limit on how long you can 'veg out'.

  Work out BEFORE you arrive at your friend's or arrange to meet another friend for a run or walk later that day (so you have to leave). And, be sure you have friends that enjoy a variety of activities...so you play video games with some, sports with some, watch movies with some...you get the idea.

Role Models...or the lack thereof

There's nothing better than a positive role model to look up to, admire and aspire to be like. Many people choose people they know and trust as role models, like parents or teachers. However, some young people don't have those positive role models in their lives. So, who do you look up to? Society and the media say...celebrities!! After all, they live the dream life and have everything you want, so it makes sense to want to be just like them. Unfortunately, some of societies chosen role models stumble and fall...or just set a really bad example...and seem to fail us. That makes it a bit confusing, especially when they seem to have great success on one hand and poor judgment on the other. On the surface it can look like bad choices don't matter if you're famous. But they do. So, please remember you need to be very careful about the people you choose to have as role models in your life.

So, how do you know how your role models stack up? First, make a list of all the people who you admire and would like to emulate (be like). It can be celebs, family members, friends and teachers...whomever you look up to. Next, you get to be a bit of an investigator. You need to find out more about these people before they are allowed on your role model list. Whether researching famous people online or asking faculty members about a fellow teacher...you want to learn how they got to where they are and how they view the world. So, here are some great questions to find answers to (some of this will come from observation):

- How they got to be where they are (their journey)?
- What things do they struggle with?
- How do they handle pressure?
- Do they have integrity and honesty?
- Is there any reason they wouldn't make a good role model?

Trisha Stewart

When you look closely at people you admire...potential role models...there are two things you need to remember. The first is that no one is perfect and everyone stumbles occasionally – the real telling thing is how they handle themselves after they've fallen a bit. The second is that if people consistently make mistakes, make poor choices and tend to blame others rather than take responsibility for themselves...they'll need to come off the list. Speaking of lists, I've included a few ideas for role models and things to keep in mind.

- **Family** – It's natural to look up to your parents, but some your people don't have their parents around them, or have parents struggling with their own issues and unable to set a good example. If you find yourself in this situation, reach further out into the family tree to aunts, uncles, cousins and grandparents until you find someone you admire and respect.
- **Friends** – We often set our friends up on a pedestal because we think so much of them. The challenge here is that it's not easy to stay on that perch (in other words they'll make a mistake and fall down in your eyes). And, some people don't want to be there and aren't comfortable being looked up to. Remember that just because someone is popular, doesn't mean they're a role model. So, select friends and peers who have achieved great things, seem focused and driven and are thought of well by others.

- **Teachers/Trainers/Coaches** - Experts and educators can make great role models. However you need to be sure they walk their talk and can be supportive of your dreams. The great thing is that because you likely have more than one teacher or coach…you can find someone who's the right role model for you!
- **Celebrities** - From actors in films to singers in concert to pro athletes hitting the field, celebrities are default role models. Because they captivate our attention and their every move seems to be caught on camera we have constant exposure to them. We see their great lives and dream of the day we'll live the same way. However, some celebrities have a public persona and a personal life that don't match up. Be sure you're looking up to celebs that have integrity and consistently positive behaviors (or handle scandal and rumors well).

Trisha Stewart

> *Don't get yourself in certain circumstances or instances, because it's not a good feeling to be sitting in that chair where you've got 12 people that are in control of your life. You have an opportunity to be in control of your life for yourself by the decisions that you make. I think that's good that I have to watch how I act and what I say. I think that's a part of growing up.*
> **P. Diddy Combs**

Stress, Fear and Loathing

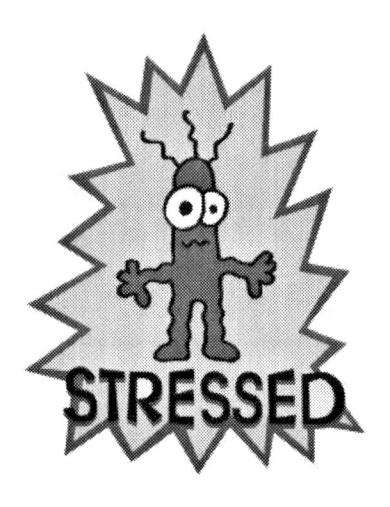

When you've got a big dream that you're working towards, you can face a great deal of stress in making sure you're hitting your goals, staying focused and doing everything you need to get done. Plus you want to be healthy, happy and well-liked. That means you can face a lot of stress on a daily basis. When you have too much stress in your life...you tend to act and react out of fear. Fear that you're not measuring up, fear of how

Healthy Idol

others will judge you, fear of failure, fear of success, and fear of change...the list goes on. That can lead to spiraling downward to a place where you not only don't trust yourself and your decisions, but you don't like yourself...a self-loathing takes over. Okay...MAJOR OBSTACLE!!! Stress happens to everyone, but the key is how to deal with it. So, let's look at how to recognize and handle it.

Believe it or not, you are in charge of your stress level. It often feels like stress happens TO YOU, but what you do have control over is how to REACT TO stressful situations. Here are some positive and healthy ways to react to stress:

- When things change or a problem arises ...don't call them problems, call them challenges. Look at the other side of the coin so to speak and find the opportunities in the situation. What can you learn or how can you grow from this?
- Identify what you CAN control or change and don't spend time worrying about those things that are beyond your control. Let those things go and keep moving.
- Take full responsibility for the way you respond to stress. In other words, do not become a victim to stress by blaming your response on the circumstances. No matter what happens, you get to choose how you will behave and respond. Napoleon Hill wrote *"You have absolute control over but one thing, and that is your*

thoughts. If you fail to control your own mind, you may be sure you will control nothing else."
- Continue to be positive about yourself. Don't let stress lead to a pessimistic or negative attitude. It helps to hang out with people who are optimistic and passionate as they can keep you up and positive. It's written somewhere, *"The pessimist complains about the wind, the optimist expects change, the realist adjusts the sails."* The wind is the challenge…who is getting the best results?
- Take great care of your body and mind…being strong and healthy helps create balance in your life and gives you the strength and ability to better handle stress.
- Have a 'letting go' outlet. A great stress reliever is to do something fun or creative…where you can let go of whatever is worrying you and just focus on what you're doing. It might be painting, writing, running or spending time with a hobby. And often times, when you set aside your worries, the solution you've been looking for will just seem to come to you.

Let's talk a little more about fear. It's said that all thoughts and actions either come from fear or from love…in other words from a positive or negative place. So, if you think about that, making a choice or decision when you're fearful is not the strongest place to be.

Healthy Idol

That means you're not likely making the best decision. Fear can shut you down, make you doubt and even make you loathe your life and who you are.

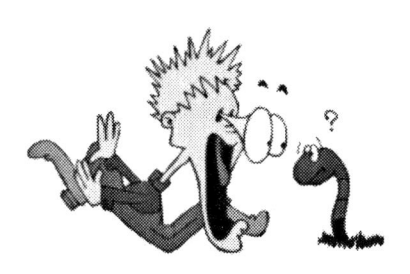

How can you expect to make the healthiest choices for yourself if that's your mindset? I'm not saying you'll never be fearful...but be aware that fear is there and try to move beyond it. Then you'll have an open mind full of creative thoughts that will help you to evolve and reach your ultimate goals.

So, Trisha...you're asking...how can I live without fear? Well, children do it. Have you ever noticed how small children just run at anything full force? They'll run straight into a swimming pool and expect to swim or onto a road and expect to cross safely or up to almost anyone and expect a hug.

That zest for life, that confidence that everything will always be okay is amazing. What happens is that as you grow you're held back. And, as far as running into a pool or out into the street...that's a good thing. We need to understand how to be safe. But, what most often happens is we're made more than just aware of dangers but taught to be fearful of them...even fearful of challenges or change.

Family and friends often share their fears with us and we end up taking them on as our own. Fear speaks up in ways you may not initially recognize as fear. These are a few things you might hear as you pursue your *Healthy Idol* dreams:

- We've always done it this way.
- It's been good enough this long, why consider changing?
- No one's ever done that before.
- What you're saying probably won't work.
- Don't rock the boat...leave things the way they are.
- That sounds impossible.
- What if you don't succeed...maybe you shouldn't try.

Obstacles are out there, but you can overcome them. If you stay focused on your goals, keep yourself strong and healthy and move beyond your fears...you will succeed.

It's like Henry Ford said, "Whether you think you can or you think you can't, you're right."

Chapter 7

Get it Right...Get Support

"Fame is a bitch, man. Success is a beast. And it actually puts the emphasis on the wrong thing. You get away with more instead of looking within." Brad Pitt

Wow! If Brad Pitt thinks fame is tough...then what must it be like for the rest of Hollywood? Sounds like he's saying it can take over your life and turn you upside down a bit. So...the road to fame is not necessarily paved in gold. That would be nice though, wouldn't it? You could just pick up a few bricks along the road to pay your way. Well, golden road fantasies aside, you will need some support to get to where you want to go. And you'll have choices to make along the way. Some will seem obvious, but others... well here are some tips for making the best choices you can along your journey.

Make the right choices

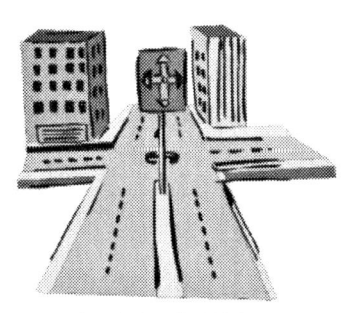

' CHOOSE RIGHT DIRECTION '

How do you know if you're making the right choices? It's not always easy. Many times you'll just have to trust yourself and your 'gut instinct' that you're making the decision that's best for you. But that instinct comes over time and even adults have decisions they struggle over...asking what's best? What's the right choice?

If you're facing some tough decisions...especially those relating to your big dreams...take some time to think about things. Don't ever feel like you have to make a decision right there on the spot. And, sometimes just taking a moment to pause can help you step back from the emotions of the situation, so you can look at things more objectively. In other words, it's okay to 'sleep on it!'

Once you've allowed yourself some time to think about your decision, you need to get all the information you can about what your choice may mean to you. A list of 'pros' and 'cons' is a good way to look at both sides of something. Just grab a piece of paper and write down the positive and negative sides to your decision.

Seeing things in writing will help you see them more clearly and make a better informed decision. Remember that it's not just about the number of 'pros' and 'cons' on your list, but how important they are to you. A decision may only have one negative consequence, but it may be something that affects

Healthy Idol

your life forever. So, no matter how many 'pros' are written down, it's just not worth risking the one negative.

It's wise to talk about big decisions with someone you can trust. Remember in Chapter 6 about finding the right role models? Sit down with that trusted parent, teacher or friend and listen to their point of view, bounce your ideas off them and be open to what they have to say. Sometimes someone else sees things in a completely different way that you do and it can be very eye opening.

Do your best to gather information and make the best decision you can, based on what you know. Once you've made your choice...keep moving forward. No one is perfect and at some point you may question a choice you've made. You might find yourself saying "Well if I'd known THAT before, I would have made a different decision." That's okay...everyone has faced that scenario. But, you can't wallow in choices you've already made or feel bad about things you didn't know. That can bog you down and keep you from making future decisions. So, you have to remind yourself that you made the best decision you could at the time.

Some choices will still be hard and sometimes you won't know for quite some time if you really did make the best decision. But, if you follow the approach I've described for you, you can be sure you're heading in the right direction. Remember:

- Gather all the information you can
- List the pros and cons
- Talk it over with someone you trust
- Make the decision based on what you know
- Move onward and upward

Have a Plan B

Have you ever heard the saying, "Don't put all your eggs in one basket"? That's what having a Plan B is about. It's clear that if you put all your fragile eggs in one basket and something happens to that basket...all the eggs are ruined. So, what does that mean in relation to you pursuing big dreams of fame and fortune? It means you need to have a broad vision of success and other options available to you.

You may not always be able to do the one thing you want to do right now. Can an athlete play basketball forever? Do supermodels work into their 40s and 50s? The answer is no, they don't. But, smart celebrities and successful people have a Plan B...a fall back business or venture where they put some of their eggs. Why do you think so many singers have perfume or clothing lines? Why do actors open up their own production studios? Why do good musicians also work as producers? It's all Plan B!!!

Healthy Idol

So, right now you're focusing on discovering and developing your true talents. That's great, but don't forget that you may need to develop other talents in order to thrive and survive. Make developing your Plan B ideas a part of your goals. You may need to go back and revisit the SMART goals you set and add to them.

If you want to be a rock star, you need to know more than how to play a guitar and sing...you need some savvy business skills. Or, you may have another passion you'd like to pursue as well...like actors and athletes who develop clothing lines. So, on your way to your ultimate goal here are some Plan B things to consider:

- **Get an Education** - First and foremost...finish high school - that's a must. And, you should consider college or some other continuing education. You may think you don't need an education, because you've already got the talent to be the next great actor, singer, dancer or athlete. Well, believe me...if nothing else...you'll need to know how to manage the people that will want to manage you! A basic education is vital...that way you can do whatever you need to along the way. I mean, how are you going to support yourself while you're waiting for your big break? Might as well have some marketable skills that get you a better paying job than delivering pizzas or newspapers, right?

- **Maintain your Health and Fitness** – Of course, that's the main focus of the ***Healthy Idol*** book...getting and keeping you healthy and strong. But part of your Plan B is to make sure you've got the stamina to keep going...even when things get tough. And who knows, maybe you'll end up with an interest in health and fitness that can be a part of your Plan B.
- **Learn the Business Side of Your Passion** – Whether it's how film studios operate, what it takes to run a record label, or how to deal with the media...having knowledge about the business side of your dream industry is vital to long-term success. There are horror stories out there on how talented but trusting people have been taken advantage of and been left with nothing. Don't let that happen to you!
- **Get a hobby** – Sure it's a great stress reliever as I mentioned in Chapter 6, but it's more than that. Hobbies can become fall back plans. For example, I know of a 'personal trainer' whose clients included entertainers and business moguls. This 'personal trainer decided to pick up a camera for fun and take some pictures. Now he has 'showings' at local galleries and does professional photo shoots.

What's something you've always wanted to try? You never know where it will lead and worst case scenario...you'll have some fun.

Healthy Idol

Realize that having a Plan B does NOT mean you doubt your ability to make it in your chosen profession. It just means you're being smart about your future and taking things into your own hands to ensure your success. So, take control and make yourself the best and most versatile **Healthy Idol** around!

Don't go it alone

> "I think the reason I never ended up in as much trouble as Paris or Lindsay seem to is that I'm not stupid, so I'd never do a lot of the things those girls do, and I've always had good friends around me. They should surround themselves with better people who don't let them get themselves in trouble. You'll never read a story about me going out and partying when I'm supposed to be working. Nor would I show up on a set drunk or miss a day's work - never."
> **Tara Reid**

Wait a minute, didn't I just say take control and take things into your own hands? Yes I did, but I didn't say you need to walk by yourself as you do it. We all need support, so surround yourself with people who care and believe in you!

Getting the right kind of support will actually help you to build your confidence. And, those people whom you trust, admire and respect will encourage you to move forward towards your chosen goal. You need to hear "Well done" when you've achieved a target...even a small one. You deserve a pat on the back when you've mastered a new skill, been cast in a show or booked an interview. Remember from Chapter 6 to be aware of those people who are not good role models or who are jealous. If you find yourself with too many of those types in your life, and not enough fans and encouragers...it's time to reach out and make new contacts.

That may feel a bit overwhelming. You may feel that you don't know anyone who is even on the same wavelength as you are, and so could never find someone to support your dreams. Well, here's your first challenge...I challenge you to get outside of your normal sphere of friends and meet some new people.

You'll find some people who share your passion, and you'd be surprised at how many of them are thrilled to share their knowledge and support you. So, make a list...go on, do it now....of all the potential supporters, friends, family, mentors, colleagues and authority figures you have contact with (or someone can introduce you to). Next, write up a little essay or summary of what you want to say about your dreams and goals...keep it brief. And, think of a few really good things you can ask them to help you with. Here are some ideas:

- I would like to appear on TV in American Idol or Dancing with the Stars or another talent show. Can you help me find the right person to talk to?

Healthy Idol

- I would like to sing some songs I have written which I would like to record for a world class recording studio. Would you mind listening to them and giving your opinion?
- I want to open a chain of health shops. Can we brainstorm some ideas so that I can make a presentation to the bank?
- I would really like to become a great professional basketball player. Would you help me figure out the best college to start my career?
- I would like to learn how to dance. Can you help me?

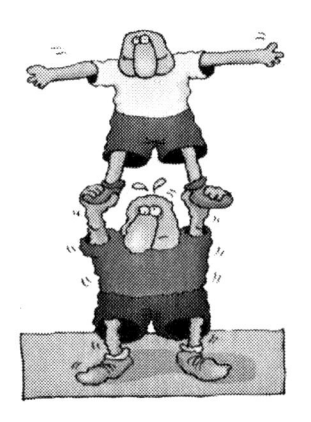

People love to support other people, so once you start asking around, I guarantee you'll find people who want to nurture, mentor and encourage you. So, when you have selected your support team, share your vision with them. Once they know your big vision, they can better help you attain your goals along the way. They may even know someone else who can help in ways they cannot. Plus, speaking your dreams out to others helps make them real in your mind. The more real they become in your mind, the greater chance that you will be successful in making that vision a reality.

Remember how I talked about visualizing yourself as a successful Healthy Idol in Chapter 1? You can do that same thing with your support team. I mean, put your cards on the table and let them know your wildest dreams.

Do you know that you want to be the next James Bond girl? Do you want to win American Idol? Do you want to play in the World Series? What will your life be like? Describe what you imagine to your support team from the clothes you'll wear to the car you'll drive (or be driven in) to the people you'll be rubbing elbows with. Name them all and make it all real so that your support team can't help but see it too...that way they can better support you on the way to making those dreams come true.

Sometimes, even with a great support team and lots of fans and admirers...it gets hard. You falter and think about giving up. Or, maybe you're still struggling to put together a support team and feel a bit too alone. It can be hard to keep positive and keep believing in yourself when things are tough. Don't forget that you can always reach out to me and my team for support as well. Just visit www.TrishaStewart.com and check

Healthy Idol

out encouraging articles, new tips and other things that will help keep you on track.

Another great idea it to have a list of positive affirmations you can read to yourself. It may sound a bit corny if you've never done this before, but trust me - it works! You can even record them so you can play them on your iPod as you're out getting your daily exercise. Here are some suggestions...but feel free to make up your own:

- I accept problems as challenges, this is how I will develop
- I see things through to their positive conclusions
- I make decisions and accept the consequences of my actions
- I accept complete responsibility for my own well-being
- I do not criticize myself, nor do I accept others negative judgment of me
- I get great satisfaction from doing my work really well
- I discipline myself through my thoughts, desires, images and expectations
- I avoid comparing myself to others in a negative way, that lowers my self esteem
- I do not let others talk me into things that I myself do not agree with or value
- I love myself
- I believe in myself and my talents

Trisha Stewart

- I will become successful...I determine my own success

Being a *Healthy Idol* will take some work and commitment on your part. But this book will help along the way as you achieve your dreams and goals. Everyone wants success and everyone wants to be happy, but you're in a position to achieve these things. You already have a talent you're developing...and now you're envisioning where that talent will take you. You've got the tools to set your goals and become a healthy strong person living their dream. Consider me a member of your support team...I believe in you and am pulling for you to make it big! See you in the spotlight!

Afterword

Well, if you've made it all the way through this book that means you're determined to go after your dreams...congratulations. But your work is just starting...getting healthy is the first half, staying healthy is the second half. It really comes down to attitude and how badly you want your dreams to come true. If you've got talent and you follow the guidelines I've laid out for you...you're well on your way to stardom (or whatever 'dom' it is you'd like to achieve).

And, remember – I'm not leaving you behind just because you're reading the last pages of this book. Visit my website, www.trishastewart.com to get ongoing motivation and support...we're always adding something new for you to check out...new articles, exercises, tips, recipes and we'll be debunking a few health and fitness myths along the way too. So, if you have a question, need some advice or just need inspiration to stay on track...see me online. If you don't find the answers you're looking for – email me and I'll get back to you with the answer.

And, be sure to keep an eye out for the "Healthy Bunch Cook Book" and "Healthy Fitness Central" to keep you eating and moving in the right way. Remember, success isn't about how big your paycheck is, how many fans you have or even what you do for a living.

Success is about you - and feeling good about who you are and how you're living your life. So, no matter what your dreams and passions...no matter if you end up in the spotlight or behind the scenes...no matter if the paparazzi ever chase you down the street...you have a Healthy Idol inside you waiting to get out. So, go for it!

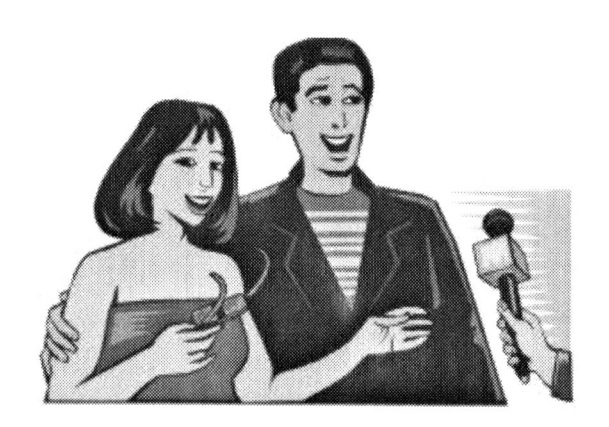

Fact File - A

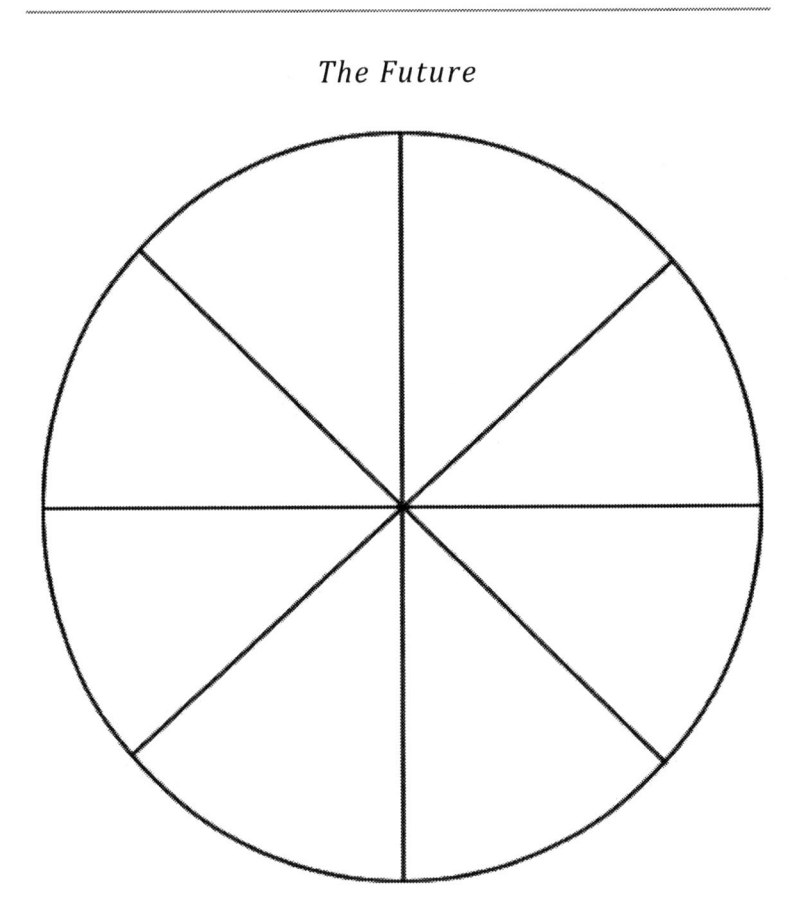

The Future

This is the wheel of your future, by filling in the segments you will see how balanced your future looks; it will probably have some high scores in some segments and low in others.

The low scores will indicate some work to do in these areas. The high scores mean you will be able to draw on these to help you balance out the low scores.

Complete the above sections with your visions as follows:

- Know what you want
- Short Term
- Medium
- Long Term
- Written Plans
- Visualization
- Resources

Number each section 1-10 with 1 being the centre – 10 being the outside of the wheel.

- **Know what you want**
  You can't have a vision if you don't know what you want, so get this in first. Be honest, is this a 1 or 10 or somewhere in between?
- **Short Term Vision**
  This could be the next 90 days. Have you planned the weeks with what you are going to achieve in them. Mark this on a 1-10 and be honest because otherwise the weeks will be gone by and you will not have even started.
- **Medium Term Vision**
  Can you visualize the next 1-5 years, I know this sounds like forever but it will soon pass, even quicker if you have not achieved any of your dreams. What plans have you in place for 1 year even – mark this 1-10 and if you are at No 1 you really need to get visualizing and planning

- **Long Term Vision**
  This will be 5+ years - wow! That's like a really long time and you are asking: Why should I be thinking that far ahead? Because you will not achieve your long term goals if you don't. Write down some of your long term visions and then mark the chart 1-10 - so, do you need to work on this?
- **Written Plans**
  Have you got these plans down, short, medium and long term? Are they in your diary or on a timeline? Do you have a prosperity chart on the wall (this is a picture of you in the middle with pictures all around you of what you are going to achieve)?
- **Visualization**
  Look into this and visualize your end result - smell it, feel it, hear it, touch it.
- **Resources**
  Have you resourced your vision? Do you have the right people supporting you? Do you have the energy?

Trisha Stewart

Fact File B

Shopping List

This shopping list is by no means extensive as I have only included really healthy ingredients. If you buy some of the ingredients, especially the dried or store cupboard goods you will always have ingredients you can pull out and throw a meal together for your hungry mates! Buying fresh ingredients on the day is best but not always possible.

You don't need to buy everything here, just work out what you need, what tastes in food you have, i.e. spicy, herby, Italian, Mexican, Chinese and so on.

Check all labels to ensure you are avoiding additives, bad carbs, saturated fats and too much salt, buy organic and what is in season wherever possible.

If your age group means a parent takes care of shopping then help out and go shopping too, it means you can be doubly sure of getting in the kind of food that will be healthy for everyone.

Enjoy your shopping and cooking adventure

- Rice Crackers, Oat Cakes, Corn Crackers (*or make your own, much tastier*)

Healthy Idol

- Porridge Oats/Oatmeal, Millet, Quinoa *(Pronounced "Keen Wa")*, Buckwheat, Bulghur Wheat, Wholegrain Rice *(Basmati Is Good But Try Wild Rice Also)*
- Lentils, (Green, Red, Brown, Puy) , Chick Peas, Mung Beans, Black Turtle Beans, Black Eyed Beans, Kidney Beans, Flageolet Beans, Haricot Beans, Pinto Beans, Butter Beans. *(all beans may be bought in cans but check no sugar/salt, cheaper to do your own from dried and don't forget you can sprout these, check www.trishastewart.com)*
- Yeast Free Stock-Marigold Swiss Bouillon is good, make sure it is low salt
- Corn Flour, Rice Flour, Potato Flour, Soya Flour *(if you are going to do a lot of cooking/baking the different types of flour are useful)*
- Rice Noodles, Rice Pasta or Corn Pasta
- Herbs *(dried are ok but fresh where possible for better flavor)*
- Spices *(will be dried in powder or seeds, use seeds where possible)*
- Seaweeds, Nori, Wakame, Kombu, Dulse, Arame, Hijiki, Agar Agar, Laver
- Shitake and Porcini dried mushrooms *(check my website for details of how to use these and the seaweeds)*

- Tamari Sauce, Piri Piri, Balsamic Vinegar, Cider Vinegar, Tahini, *(check those labels for too much salt and buy organic or the best quality)*
- Extra Virgin Olive Oil, Canola Oil, Sesame Oil, Walnut Oil, Coconut oil, (buy cold pressed and organic oils where possible) Coconut Milk/Cream
- Canned Tomatoes (ok if fresh not available, check no sugar/salt)
- Sunflower, Pumpkin, Sesame, Hemp, Flax/Linseeds *(great snacks and you can sprout them if you like or make into seed butters)* Almonds, Brazil Nuts, Macadamia, Cashew and Hazelnuts, *(great for nut butters as well as snacks)*
- Black Pepper, Rock Salt *(salt minimum use)*, Mustard Powder
- Fresh chilies, ginger, garlic
- Fresh vegetables/salads and fruit, carrots, swede, turnips, parsnip, kohlrabi, sweet potato, squash/pumpkin, beetroot (beets), onions, garlic, scallions, shallots, artichokes, cabbage red/green/white, spinach, kale, broccoli, brussel sprouts, cauliflower, asparagus, swiss chard, green beans. Various herb leaves, lettuce, cucumber, courgette (zucchini), peppers, celery, aubergine (eggplant) and so much more.... *(go for it and try something you have not had before)*

Healthy Idol

- Lemons and Limes *(sliced added to hot water or for salad dressings)*
- Tofu (great low fat, high protein, lots of uses, scramble, marinate, stew, layer up)
- Hummus, Guacamole, (or buy the fresh ingredients and make your own)
- Rice Milk, Soya (Soy) Milk or Nut Milk (see recipes to make your own)
- Soya (Soy) Yoghurt
- Eggs, Chicken, Fish, Meat, *(be so aware of the reasons for buying organic or not eating this at all)*
- Feta, Cottage, Ricotta, Haloumi, Goats Cheeses *(ditto)*

Trisha Stewart

Fact File C

Juices, Smoothies & Recipes

- ✓ Healthy Idol's need juice and smoothies
- ✓ Each recipe is enough for one serving
- ✓ Blend ice cubes or serve over ice if liked

As I am not sure of your age because this book is for a wide age group you may not be into cooking but I am sure you can all make a smoothie or a juice and nut or seed butter but make sure you clean up afterwards !

Juices

Get up and Go

- o 2 apples preferably those which will give lots of juice, royal gala, pink lady, golden delicious or your preference
- o ¼ pineapple
- o Half a small lime or ¼ lemon or a bit of each
- o ½ avocado (put a little lemon juice on the other half to stop it going brown
- o Small piece of cucumber or courgette / zucchini
- o Handful of parsley
- o Put everything but the avocado through the juicer
- o Blend the avocado and mix together

Healthy Idol

Reviver

- Two apples
- ½ small carrot or ¼ large one
- ½ small beetroot (beet) or ¼ large one
- Broccoli floret
- Bunch of mixed greens including spinach and parsley
- Small piece of courgette / zucchini or cucumber
- Small piece of celery (if liked as it can sometimes overrule the flavor)
- Small piece of ginger (to taste)
- ¼ lemon
- Sprouts such as alfalfa

Put all the ingredients through the juicer and enjoy

Snack Attack (1)

- Two apples
- 1 carrot
- Bunch of mixed greens
- Piece celery
- ½ lemon
- ¼ cucumber

Put it all through the juicer

Snack Attack (2)

- ¼ Pineapple
- ½ avocado
- ¼ lime
- Small piece of Ginger
- Two apples

Put all, except the avocado through the juicer, blend the avocado and mix together and drink.

Earthy but lush

- Bunch of greens (spinach, kale, broccoli, cabbage etc)
- Small bunch parsley
- ¼ beetroot
- two apples
- 1 carrot
- Small piece of celery

Put all through the juicer

Basically carrots, apples and greens make great juices, a daily juice to include apples, carrots and celery would be great a great combo but add more to taste.

All the juices are packed full of vitamins, minerals, bioflavonoids and real live enzymes you just can't go wrong with your choice.

It is worth adding wheatgrass!

1. Purifies and alkalizes the blood
2. Helps prevent or reverse constipation
3. Stimulates the liver
4. Helps to rid the body of toxins
5. Increases enzyme activity in the digestive system
6. Helps to increase the level of good bacteria in the gut
7. Helps the kidneys to cleanse and detoxify

If you are going to add wheatgrass my advice is to take it as a "shot" in a 1fl oz shot glass and have a little ginger added or a ¼ orange to suck afterwards. It does overpower other juice ingredients so it may ruin what would have been a tasty juice for you. Experiment and find out what works best for you.

Healthy Idol

Grow your own wheatgrass as well as sprouts

Take a couple of handfuls of wheatgrass and put through the juicer, it is fabulous to look at so bright and invigorating.

Smoothies

Use frozen fruit that has been defrosted for a few minutes as this will make a lovely thick shake or blend with ice cubes.

Berry Delight

1 cup of banana

½ cup each of berries such as strawberries, raspberries, blackberries or blueberries and blend with a little honey or maple syrup and ice if berries not frozen

Whizz up in the blender

Mango Madness

- 1 cup mango
- 2 cups fresh squeezed orange juice
- ¼ cup pitted dates
- Small handful of seeds (flax, sunflower, pumpkin or whatever is available, grind in a coffee grinder)
- 1 small banana
- If fruits not frozen blend with ice cubes

Caribbean Smooch

- ¼ cup each of banana, berries, mango, pineapple, papaya, fresh coconut and ¼ cup of its water

Whizz up in a blender and enjoy....

Nut Butter Smoothie

- ½ cup banana, berries (or mango, pineapple)
- 1 tablespoon of nut butter (see recipes)

Whizz up in the blender and drink lots of nutrients

Carob Cocktail

- 2-3 tablespoons of raw carob powder
- ½ cup each of banana, berries or mango
- ¼ cup coconut flesh (chopped)
- 1 tablespoon honey or maple syrup

Whizz up and drink

Nut Butters

- Two cups of your favorite nuts such as cashews, macadamia, walnuts, almonds (soak overnight or for a few hours and remove any skins)
- ½ cup of apple, orange or other juice

Grind the nuts in a processor, add the liquid and hey presto! a delicious and nutritious butter to add to smoothies, spread onto oatcakes or use any way you wish.

You can do the same with seeds such as pumpkin, sesame, sunflower etc.

Healthy Idol

Breakfasts

Here again, depending on age group, you may be able to prepare some of these yourself, go on, give it a try, get everyone's breakfast by making up a batch of porridge or muesli. But, get permission or help to make the other recipes if necessary.

Porridge (Oatmeal)

This can be a simple cupful of oats to 3 or 4 cups of water or a mix of water and some kind of milk. Put in a small pan, just bring to simmer for a few minutes, add more fluid if necessary. It will depend on the oats as to how much fluid.

You can make millet or quinoa porridge in exactly the same way but may need to vary the fluid

Or make a mix of oats, millet and quinoa.

You can add to this the following:

1. Pure vanilla essence or a vanilla pod
2. Nutmeg
3. Cinnamon
4. Nuts and Seeds, ground or whole
5. Fresh stewed fruit
6. A little soya (soy) yoghurt

Muesli

1 cup of each of rice flakes and millet. Add chopped nuts, sunflower seeds, sesame seeds, pumpkin seeds and flax seeds. Soak in soya or rice milk for half an hour or less -if you like the mixture a little dry then top with soya (natural) yoghurt

Trisha Stewart

Healthy Cookies

Oatcakes

- 350gm of fine oatmeal or coarse if you like a rustic oatcake
- 1 tsp of good quality rock salt
- 150ml pint boiling water
- 50 ml of olive oil, walnut or other oil (may need to check consistency and add more) you can also use tahini, nut butter or any vegan butter that will melt.
- Pinch of bicarbonate of soda

Mix everything together and turn out onto a board, knead and roll out into two big rounds. Make some cuts across to form triangles and bake on a tray which has been oiled.

Bake in a cool oven of around 150c (300f) or gas mark 2 for about one hour, do not overcook or they will be too hard.

You can add other ingredients to flavor, sweet or savory, such as sun dried tomatoes, herbs, garlic, ginger or cinnamon, nutmeg, vanilla and so on....experiment....

How about making some Hummus to dip your oatcakes into?

Ingredients

225g/8oz chick peas	canned without salt or sugar or dried, soaked overnight and cooked until soft
3 cloves garlic	crushed
2 lemons	juiced

Healthy Idol

150ml/5floz tahini

50ml/2floz olive oil

To garnish, olive oil, paprika and chopped parsley

Preparation

Put all the ingredients except garnish into a blender and whizz up till smooth, you may need to add more lemon juice or water to get the consistency you like.

Put into a serving dish and garnish

When blending, you can add roasted red peppers or other roasted vegetables or pesto.

Soups

Soups can be anything added to the pot so that you get a great tasty meal but I have listed a couple of recipes below so that you can work from the basics of these - be adventurous with your cooking, where I have listed measurements for the ingredients, get used to a handful of this and a handful of that, taste as you go and get those senses working.

Carrot and Coriander

Ingredients (serve 6)

1 tbs Olive or sunflower oil

450g/1lb Carrots   washed and chopped

350g/12oz leeks   washed and chopped

1 tbsp coriander seeds	roasted in a frying pan, then lightly crushed using a pestle and mortar or wrap the seeds in some greaseproof paper and crush
½ Lemon	Use the zest (grate the skin) and 1 tbsp juice

900ml/1 ½ pint vegetable stock or yeast free bouillon

Fresh ground pepper to taste

Preparation

Gently fry the leeks and carrots in the oil for 15 minutes until vegetables almost soft

Stir in coriander seeds and lemon zest and fry for 2-3 minutes

Add stock and bring to the boil, simmer for 10 minutes

Cool soup slightly, liquidize until smooth

Return to pan, add lemon juice, black pepper warm through and add some fresh chopped coriander to garnish

This recipe works well with sweet potato, parsnip, celeriac, onions or garlic.

Tomato Soup

Ingredients (serves 6)

2 tbsp	Sunflower or olive oil
1 Clove Garlic	crushed
1 med onion	chopped small

Healthy Idol

700g/1 ½ lb fresh tomatoes	blanched, peeled and coarsely chopped

1 tsp maple syrup or honey

625ml/1pt vegetable stock, yeast free bouillon or fresh made

1 tbsp fresh basil	chopped

Fresh ground black pepper to taste

Preparation

Gently fry the onions and garlic in the oil for 10 minutes

Add tomatoes and honey/maple syrup a cook for 1 minute

Add stock and bring to the boil, turn down and simmer for 15 minutes, at the end of this add the fresh basil

Cool slightly and put into a liquidizer: blend until smooth

Put back into pan, heat slowly, add black pepper to taste

You can add lentils or haricot beans to this for a hearty soup and if there is any leftover you can make a base for a lasagna, chili or curry. You can add the sauce to vegetables and serve with some whole grains, pasta and a salad or other side dishes.

Curried Parsnip Soup

Ingredients (serve 4-6)

2 tbsp sunflower, olive or coconut oil

1 onion	sliced
675g/1 ½ lbs parsnips	washed, thinly peeled and diced

Trisha Stewart

5ml/1 ½ tsp curry powder
(you could use a paste if you have one)

2.5ml/1/2 tsp ground cumin

1200ml/2pts vegetable stock, yeast free bouillon or fresh made

150ml/1/4pt soya milk, rice milk or coconut milk

Fresh black pepper to taste

Paprika to garnish

Preparation

Gently fry onion and chopped parsnips in the oil

Add curry powder and ground cumin and cook gently for a further 2 minutes.

Add the stock and bring to boil, turn down and simmer until the vegetables are cooked, approx 15 minutes.

Cool soup slightly and put into a liquidizer and blend until smooth.

Return to the saucepan and add the milk and black pepper, heat through.

Garnish with parsley and a sprinkling of paprika.

This soup could be made as spicy as you like. Other vegetables could be used instead or in addition to parsnips such as sweet potato, carrots, celeriac and Jerusalem artichokes. This could also be used as a sauce over cooked vegetables with a mashed potato topping and put under the grill (non meat shepherd's pie)

Healthy Idol

How about some burgers with a difference?

Tofu and Bean Burgers

Makes 6-8

- 1 medium onion, peeled and chopped
- 1 large peeled garlic clove or to taste
- 1 medium carrot, peeled and coarsely grated (about 60g prepared weight)
- 420g can 'no-salt no-sugar' red kidney beans, drained and rinsed in a colander under cold running water or a mix of other beans
- 220g pack smoked or natural tofu, drained
- 75g/ cup sunflower seeds
- 1 small bunch parsley (about 20g)
- 2 tsp organic wheat and yeast free vegetable bouillon powder

Preparation

Preheat the oven to 220C (430f). Line a large baking tray with baking parchment. Place all the ingredients in a food processor and blend: do not puree. If you don't have a food processor, crumble or mash the tofu and beans and add to the other ingredients.

Grab a handful of mixture and form into a ball and place on the baking tray. Press with fingertips to make a burger shape, how many you will get depends on the size burger you would like. Bake for 25 minutes, do not overcook, these are great hot or cold or served with a creamy sauce, potato wedges and a salad.

Bean Casserole

- 2 large onions sliced

- Little olive oil
- 2 cloves garlic diced (or to taste)
- 1" piece of ginger sliced or diced
- 4 Tomatoes sliced
- ½ Courgette/Zucchini sliced
- 4 tbs Tahini
- 500ml vegetable stock from yeast free bouillon or homemade stock
- Mixed beans such as Haricot, Kidney, Flageolet, Butter (cooked) if using tinned ensure sugar and salt free and rinse thoroughly
- 2 tsp mixed dried herbs such as Italian or Provence
- 1 Large Sweet Potato sliced

Preparation

- In a large sauté pan, put a little olive oil and saute the sliced onions till translucent
- Add the garlic and ginger saute for a minute or two
- Add the tomatoes and courgettes
- Add the beans
- Mix the tahini, herbs and vegetable stock and add to the mixture, do not make it too wet at this stage
- Put into a casserole dish
- Place the sweet potato on top
- Bake in the oven on 170c (325f) gas 3 for about an hour

You can leave it all in the sauté pan, put the potato on top and simmer with a lid on, baked in the oven is nicer though.

You may need to add a little stock if the casserole gets to look dry.

This is a great casserole to have when the weather is a little cooler or an evening when the sun has gone down, add some side salads and some friends and you have a great night in.

Healthy Idol

Tabbouleh

- 1 cup of bulgur wheat
- 1 ½ cups of boiling water
- 3 tbsp lemon juice
- 1 clove garlic grated or crushed in a pestle and mortar
- Bunch of fresh mint chopped or ½ tsp dried
- ¾ tbsp olive oil
- 4/6 spring onions chopped (use the green if nice)
- 3 tomatoes diced
- 1 small cucumber diced
- ½ cup of olives if liked
- Bunch parsley some chopped some left for garnish

Preparation

- Combine the bulgar wheat and water, stir and let sit for 30 minutes to re-hydrate.
- Stir after the 30 minutes to check there is no moisture, if there is drain off.
- Add lemon juice, garlic and oil.
- Add the remaining ingredients and stir.

This is nice if left to sit for a while so that the flavors can combine.

This is a great dish to share with friends: add some side dishes such as lots of raw vegetable sticks or put the tabbouleh into crunchy salad leaves and eat with your fingers.

The following recipe you will do again and again, it is so tasty and versatile: eat on its own with some naan bread or pita bread and salads or as a side dish to curry.

Red Lentil Dhal

- Olive oil
- 1 tsp garlic, crushed

- 1 tsp each fresh chili and ginger, finely chopped and mixed
- 2 tsp powdered turmeric
- 3 tsp garam masala
- 3 tsp ground coriander
- 2 tbsp fresh coriander, finely chopped
- 1 cinnamon stick
- 2 tsp mustard
- 1 large whole tomato, diced finely
- 1 medium onion, diced finely
- 2 sticks celery, diced finely
- 2L/3½pt water
- 1kg/2¼lb red lentils, washed well

Preparation

- Heat the oil in a saucepan with a thick base
- Add garlic, chili, ginger and spices (except fresh coriander) and herbs, mustard, tomato, onion and celery.
- Fry for about 10 minutes until well blended.
- Add the water and bring to the boil
- Stir the lentils in and cook on a low heat for about half an hour, until the lentils are soft, stirring occasionally.

You may need to add a little stock or water if the dhal becomes dry.

If you have time place a couple of bulbs or garlic in the oven and roast for half an hour, take out and press the juicy roasted garlic and add to the dhal, some chopped almonds on top are nice and also the fresh coriander.

Healthy Idol

Salads

I am sure I don't need to tell you how to wash a few leaves and slice up some raw veggies – but here are some dressings to add

Salad Dressings

Oriental
- 6 tablespoons olive oil
- 2 teaspoons of lemon juice
- 4 teaspoons soy sauce
- ½ teaspoon grated root ginger put into a jar and shake.

French
- 6 tablespoons olive oil
- 2 tablespoons lemon juice
- 2 tablespoons cider vinegar.

Variations on the above could include crushed garlic, balsamic vinegar, mustard and any fresh herbs you may like.

Shake it all in a jar or put into a blender.

Soya (Soy)
Take a tub of natural soya (soy) yoghurt and put in a blender with a choice of any herbs or spices, this will make a dressing or a dip for crudités

Whizz in a blender

Tomato Dressing
- 100ml olive oil
- 2 tablespoons tomato puree or sun dried tomatoes,
- 1 teaspoon cumin, allspice, oregano, marjoram and a little cayenne pepper (vary any).

Whizz in a blender

Get the **Healthy Bunch Cookbook** for more great recipes www.healthybunchcookbook.com.

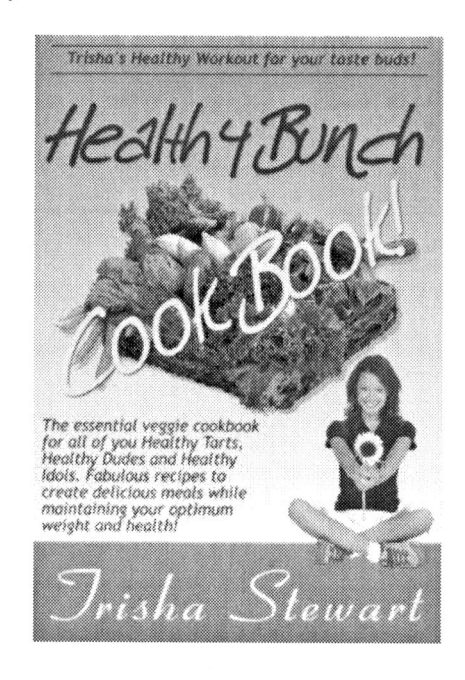

Healthy Idol

Fact File D

Fast Food

I am sure some of you have watched the movie "Supersize Me" in which Morgan Spurlock ate at McDonalds's three times daily and "supersized" each meal.

Morgan went from a fit, tall, healthy man, in thirty days, he gained 24.5lbs and a massive 13% body mass. He also suffered sexual dysfunction, mood swings and liver damage and it then took him fourteen months to lose that extra weight!!

The consequences of that film were that McDonald's changed its menu and included healthy options but also increased its range of other unhealthy foods.

You will already have read in this book in which I discuss that even the so called "healthy salads" contain a range of very unhealthy chemicals in them so there is, as I have already said, no reason at all to eat at McDonald's but do read on as there is more...

The egg's reputation is recovering since Edwina Curry caused havoc in the UK egg industry. But, read on - scrambled eggs at McDonald's include more harmful ingredients than egg. Their pasteurized whole eggs have sodium acid pyrophosphate, citric acid, and monosodium phosphate (all added to preserve color), and nisin, a preservative. The eggs and their chemical friends are prepared with liquid margarine: liquid soybean oil, water, partially hydrogenated cottonseed and soybean oils (trans fats), salt, hydrogenated cottonseed oil (trans fat), soy lecithin, mono- and diglycerides, sodium benzoate, potassium sorbate (preservatives), artificial flavor, citric acid, vitamin A palmitate, and beta carotene (color). What on earth is that all about – well of course its cheap and has a long shelf life !

And, what about a cup of coffee on the way to work ? well apart from coffee being an un-necessary stimulant this is what else you will find in that coffee: sodium phosphate, sodium polyphosphate, Di-Acetyl Tartrate Ester of Monoglyceride, sodium stearoyl lactylate, tetra sodium pyrophosphate, sodium hexametaphosphate, sodium citrate, and carrageenan. Wow, again, who needs all that stuff when all you wanted was a cup of coffee.....

Salads are usually a good bet but not at McDonald's they add some interesting ingredients. The salads with grilled chicken also have liquid margarine (trans fat).

Several salads have either cilantro lime glaze, or orange glaze, together with many of McDonald's dressings; both the cilantro lime glaze and the orange glaze contain propylene glycol alginate. While propylene glycol is considered acceptable for human consumption, it is not legal for use in cat food as it has

Healthy Idol

not been proven to be safe!! Propylene glycol is also used to kill off insects, ground beetles etc. (Check Wikipedia.org for info)

The chili lime tortilla strips included in the south west salads have ingredients which hide MSG. But, they also contain two ingredients that advertise the presence of MSG: disodium inosinate, and disodium guanylate. More chemical cocktails!

The chicken has sodium phosphates (foaming agent) but it does not say which source, it could be one of the following, trisodium phosphate (a cleanser), monosodium phosphate (a laxative), or disodium hydrogen phosphate, none sound like food to me. Why would McDonald's add sodium phosphates (a foaming agent), and then add *dimethylpolysiloxan an antifoaming agent* in their crispy chicken breast filets? Sounds like it should be in the dishwasher; which it will be in the form of soap powder!

Burger King

The ingredients list for a burger consist of six ingredients commonly used to hide free glutamate (MSG), they are: calcium caseinate, hydrolyzed corn, yeast extract, soy protein isolate, spices, and natural flavors. They also state at the end that this is not a vegan product and that it is cooked in a microwave!! I think this deserves a government health warning!!

Their menu has various salads but who is going to have a plain salad when they can have a dressing on it instead. Ken's Fat Free Ranch Dressing includes titanium dioxide (an artificial color, or sunscreen, depending on use!!), preservatives, and of course good old monosodium glutamate for taste and salt to make you thirsty!!

Even a simple chicken breast has been ruined; just look at the list of ingredients:

TENDERGRILL® CHICKEN BREAST FILET

Chicken Breast with Rib Meat, Water, Seasoning (Maltodextrin, Salt, Sugar, Autolyzed Yeast Extract, Garlic Powder, Spices, Natural Flavors, Onion Powder, Modified Corn Starch, Chicken Fat, Chicken Powder, Chicken Broth, Disodium Guanylate and Disodium Inosinate, Citric Acid, Partially Hydrogenated Soybean Oil, Dehydrated Garlic, and Artificial Flavors.), Modified Corn Starch, Soybean Oil, Salt, Sodium Phosphates. Glazed with: Water, Seasoning [Maltodextrin, Salt, Sugar, Methylcellulose, Autolyzed Yeast Extract, Partially Hydrogenated Sunflower Oil, Modified Potato Starch, Fructose, Partially Hydrogenated Soybean Oil, Garlic Powder, Onion Powder, Dehydrated Garlic, Spices, Modified Corn Starch, Xanthan Gum, Natural Flavors,

Healthy Idol

Disodium Guanylate and Disodium Inosinate, Chicken Fat, Caramel Color, Grill Flavor (from Partially Hydrogenated Soybean and Cottonseed Oil), Chicken Powder, Chicken Broth, Turmeric, Smoke Flavor, Annatto Extract, and Artificial Flavors], Soybean Oil.

Check out www.wikipedia.com and find out all the uses for the above chemicals added into chicken – they will be used in all sorts of manufacturing, detergents, sunscreens and so on.

Shall we go on to:

Taco Bell – an all American fast food joint

Taco Bell's website did not seem to have much to say about health! The mission is to *Keep it Balanced*, a usage of words I feel. It had no serious information on how to really eat healthy. They recommend foods like pizza and tacos, Ha......

The seasoned beef, carne asada steak, spicy shredded chicken, and even the rice all include autolyzed yeast extract (hidden MSG). Disodium inosinate and disodium guanylate are flavor enhancers used in synergy with MSG. Therefore, menu items with disodium inosinate and/or disodium guanylate also contain MSG, even the healthy sounding avocado ranch dressing, southwest chicken, citrus salsa, creamy jalapeno sauce, creamy lime sauce, lime seasoned red strips, pepper jack sauce, and seasoned rice all contain MSG!

Dimethylpolysiloxane *is optically clear, and is generally considered to be inert, non-toxic, and non-flammable.* It is used in silicone caulk, adhesives, and as an anti-foaming agent. Guess what? It's also included in Taco Bell's rice.

Wendy's

Seems healthy at the outset but wait till you read on - The mandarin chicken salad, sounds healthy? It has diced chicken, mandarin oranges, almonds, crispy noodles, a choice of dressings, and five different varieties of lettuce. Check the ingredients list. The almonds are roasted and salted. The crispy noodles are not whole grain. The mandarin orange segments are not freshly peeled oranges; most likely canned. The diced chicken has added autolyzed yeast extract (MSG), disodium inosinate, disodium guanylate, sodium phosphates (soap?), salt, more salt, sugar, modified corn startch and of course spices, natural flavors and artificial flavors.

Oh and the salad dressings include titanium dioxide in the Low Fat Honey Mustard Dressing and the Reduced Fat Creamy Ranch Dressing a versatile chemical used to manufacture paint, sunscreen, semiconductors, and food coloring!

Healthy Idol

Wendy's Southwest Taco Salad is a salad with Wendy's chili. The chili has hidden MSG: autolyzed yeast extract, spices, artificial flavors, natural flavorings, disodium inosinate and disodium guanylate (MSG give-aways). Why does chili need to include an anti-caking agent such as silicon dioxide (also known as sand, or glass powder).

By now you should be able to spot the pitfalls of soap, sunscreen and the such like in the ingredients list, have a game with your friends and see who can spot the deliberate mistake!

Seasoned Tortilla Strips

Whole Corn, Vegetable Oil (contains one or more of the following: corn, soybean or sunflower oil), Salt, Buttermilk Solids, Spices, Tomato, Sweet Cream, Dextrose, Onion, Sugar, Cheddar Cheese (cultured milk, salt, enzymes), Corn Starch, Modified Corn Starch, Maltodextrin, Nonfat Dry Milk, Garlic, Torula Yeast, Citric Acid, Autolyzed Yeast, Natural and Artifical Flavor, Artificial Colors (including extractives of paprika, turmeric and annatto, titanium dioxide, red 40, yellow 5, blue 1), Disodium Phosphate, Lactic Acid, Soy Lecithin. CONTAINS: MILK.

Tasty?? I think not...

I guess I should include KFC

Trisha Stewart

Kentucky Fried Chicken

The list of chemicals for KFC is endless, with such an extensive menu!

The chicken, the gravy, and even the rice all have monosodium glutamate added so of course the chicken in the salads also has MSG. The "healthy option" House Side Salad without dressing has nothing more than iceberg lettuce, romaine lettuce, and tomatoes.

KFC claims 0g trans fat per serving for all their fried chicken. But The Extra Crispy Chicken, Colonel's Crispy Strips, HBBQ Wings, Boneless HBBQ Wings, Fiery Buffalo Wings, and more have partially hydrogenated soybean oil listed in the ingredients. So if the trans fat content is below 0.5g per serving, they can round down to zero and claim zero grams per serving, very clever!

Check out the long list of chemical ingredients on my website www.trishastewart.com or even better go onto theirs it is open for the public to view.

My view is if you can't pronounce, it spell it or understand what it is – don't eat it!

- www.kfc.com
- www.mcdonalds.com

Healthy Idol

- www.subway.com
- www.wendys.com
- www.burgerking.com
- www.tacobell.com

Plus there are many additional sites you can check out, don't become obsessed just get healthy the natural way.

Trisha Stewart

Fact File E

Drugs

There are very many types of "substances" available to anyone who is interested. These drugs are illegal in some cases and under prescription in others; they are harmful either in the short or the long term.

They come in the many guises, even prescribed by your own GP, although of course not intentionally for the patient to abuse them.

The number of Americans who abuse controlled prescription drugs has nearly doubled from 7.8 million to 15.1 million from 1992 to 2003 and abuse among teens has more than tripled during that time, according to a new report by The National Center on Addiction and Substance Abuse (CASA) at Columbia University (extract from medical news today.com) These numbers are increasing daily and that is not counting the numbers of teenagers and adults administering illegal drugs, the whole situation is frightening.

Some of the Illegal Drugs

- **Marijuana - so you think this is safe? Well read on.** This drug is also known as Cannabis - its short/long term effects are:
    - Impaired short-term memory
    - Impaired attention, judgment, and other cognitive functions
    - Impaired coordination and balance
    - Increased heart rate
    - Impaired memory and learning skills

Healthy Idol

- - Hallucinations if taking massive doses
  - Can lead to addiction
  - Increased risk of chronic cough, bronchitis, and emphysema
  - Increased risk of cancer of the head, neck, and lungs

- **Inhalants**
  Glues, paint thinners, dry cleaning fluids, gasoline, felt tip pens, correction fluid, hair spray, aerosol deodorants, spray paint and so on.....

  Effects include giddiness, confusion, long term use effects are nosebleeds, headaches, loss of hearing and sense of smell.

  Other effects include muscle weakness, abdominal pain, severe mood swings and violent behavior, numbness and tingling of the hands and feet, nausea, limb spasms, fatigue, and lack of coordination
  Severe toxic reaction, even death

  You only need to do this once for any or all of the above contraindications.

- **Inhalant Statistics**

  Suffocation, inhaling fluid or vomit into the lungs, and accidents each cause about 15% of deaths linked to inhalant abuse. [1]

  Approximately 8.9% of youth ages 12–17 have misused inhalants. [2]

55% of deaths linked to inhalant abuse are caused by "Sudden Sniffing Death Syndrome." SSDS can occur on the first use or any use. [1]

22% of inhalant abusers who died of SSDS had no history of previous inhalant abuse. In other words, they were first-time users. [1]

Sources

[1] In the Know Zone
[2] US Dept. of Health & Human Services
[3] National Institute on Drug Abuse
[4] Monitoring the Future Survey

- **Hallucinogens**
  There are many different kinds of hallucinogens. Some occur naturally, in trees, vines, seeds, fungi and leaves. Others are manufactured in laboratories.

  The one thing they all have in common is they are dangerous.

  - LSD (lysergic acid diethylamide) - Acid, trips, microdots, dots.
  - magic mushrooms (psilocybin) - Shrooms, mushies, magics, golden tops, blue meanies, liberty caps
  - morning glory seeds
  - datura
  - mescaline (peyote cactus)
  - PCP (phencyclidine) - Angel dust, peace pill.
  - Ketamine - Special K, K, ket, kitkat, super K
  - ecstasy (MDMA and related drugs, in high doses)
  - cannabis (in high quantities).

Healthy Idol

These drugs are highly dangerous as they can cause violent sickness and diarrhea, panic attacks, confusion, mental disturbances, heart attack, epileptic fits and more.

- Stimulants – Adderall, Dexedrine, Ritalin (all prescription only drugs) – they are now used for ADHD and obesity and are also being abused by street users.

Other illegal stimulants include:

- Methamphetamines – Powerful Stimulant
- Amphetamines - VERY addictive - very quickly tolerated (need for more and more)
    - Resulting in restlessness, sleeplessness, paranoia and hallucinations – users can believe things such as insects crawling under the skin – prolonged use may result in violent and aggressive behavior, psychosis and permanent brain damage as well as heart attacks and epileptic fits.
    Other stimulants are cocaine/crack, ecstasy, crystal meth.
- Depressants - including drugs like heroin, opium, morphine, codeine and methadone, cannabis, sedatives and hypnotics (including valium and rohypnol) BZP (bensodiazepines) Barbiturates and other sedative/hypnotics are medically prescribed to treat sleeplessness, anxiety, and tension, and to help prevent or mitigate epileptic seizures.

These drugs are also common in date rape.
These are some of the most addictive drugs; they are medically prescribed although illegal on the street where a lot of them end up.

The effects are severe dependency; the **long-term effect** of barbiturates - particularly of protracted high-dose abuse - is not unlike a state of chronic inebriation.

Symptoms include the impairment of memory and judgment; hostility, depression, or mood swings; chronic fatigue; and stimulation of pre-existing emotional disorders, which may result in paranoia or thoughts of suicide.

Most drug users will use a combination of all of these "uppers and downers", they are very adept at preventing the ultimate "cold turkey" – (coming off drugs).

Past Month Illicit Drug Use among Persons Aged 12 or older, by Age: 2006 www.drugabusestatistics.samsha.gov

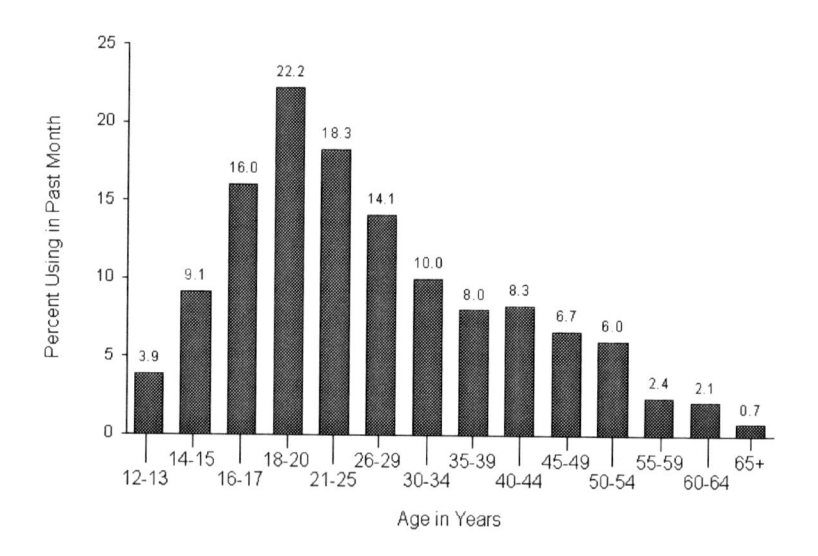

Age in Years	Percent Using in Past Month
12-13	3.9
14-15	9.1
16-17	16.0
18-20	22.2
21-25	18.3
26-29	14.1
30-34	10.0
35-39	8.0
40-44	8.3
45-49	6.7
50-54	6.0
55-59	2.4
60-64	2.1
65+	0.7

- Although adults aged 26 or older were less likely to be current drug users than youths aged 12 to 17 or young adults aged 18 to 25 (6.1 vs. 9.8 and 19.8 percent, respectively), there were more drug users aged 26 or older (11.4 million) than in the 12-to-17-year age group (2.5 million) and 18-to-25-year age group (6.5 million) combined

- **Steroids** – what are they and how are they affecting the many people that use them both legally and illegally. It is a fact that nearly 30% of 8th - 12th graders are using anabolic steroids
- **Anabolic steroids** are found naturally in our body, they are involved in our growth, physical development and reproductive organs. Prescribed or illegal, these drugs that body builders, sports persons and athletes use are man-made.

The major side effects from abusing anabolic steroids can include liver tumours and cancer, jaundice (yellowish pigmentation of skin, tissues, and body fluids), fluid retention, high blood pressure, increases in LDL (bad cholesterol), and decreases in HDL (good cholesterol). Other side effects include kidney tumours, severe acne, and trembling. In addition, there are some gender-specific side effects:

- For men - shrinking of the testicles, reduced sperm count, infertility, baldness, development of breasts, increased risk for prostate cancer.
- For women - growth of facial hair, male-pattern baldness, changes in or cessation of the menstrual cycle, enlargement of the clitoris, deepened voice.
- For adolescents - growth halted prematurely through premature skeletal maturation and accelerated puberty changes. This means that adolescents risk remaining short for the remainder of their lives if they take anabolic steroids before the typical adolescent growth spurt

Other steroids

- Some steroids occur naturally in the body, such as cortisol, sex hormones, bile acids. Cortisol is essential for all life. There are many kinds of steroids, Cortico, Glutico, Sex Hormones
- You could be using steroids and not even know it. Steroids come in various forms: shot, pill, bronchial inhalers, nasal sprays, skin creams. Steroid therapy is used for many illnesses: Ulcerative Colitis, Lupus, Severe Asthma, Rheumatic fever, Organ transplants, Allergies are only a few.

Side effects - these can be horrific and permanent

- weight gain
- hypertension
- skin atrophy (wasting away)
- myopathy (muscle disease/weakness)
- impaired wound healing
- post traumatic (after-shock) stress (anxiety, fear) suppression (lowering) of immune response (defense of body against virus, bacteria)
- subcutaneous (under skin) tissue atrophy (decrease)
- mood swings (ranging from euphoria to suicidal thoughts)
- steroid psychosis (including hallucinations, mania, delusions)
- skin infections
- depression
- hair loss
- excessive facial hair growth
- ingrown hairs
- arthritis
- coronary artery disease
- osteoporosis
- contact dermatitis
- acne, eczema
- cysts, rashes
- lesions, blisters

Healthy Idol

- open-angled glaucoma
- fatigue
- cataracts
- menstrual irregularities
- premature menopause
- secondary diabetes mellitus
- sleep disorders
- water retention
- growth retardation in children
- cushing's syndrome (affects almost every system in the body; moonface, humpback, central obesity, chronic fatigue and other symptoms)
- steroid induced asthma
- headaches
- shakiness and tremors
- easy bruising
- adhesive arachnoiditis (from epidural steroid injections)
- necrosis (a localized death of tissue) osteonecrosis
- increase susceptibility to infection
- redistribution of body fat
- increase in circulating blood fats (triglycerides)
- toxic shock
- muscle cramping, joint pain

Smoking/Nicotine

Smoking is the primary cause of cancer, everyone knows that but did you know it is as addictive as any other drug?

Smoking causes the nasal passages to become sensitive, the sinuses to become clogged which will have an effect of your ability to taste and smell.

Digestive problems such as acid reflux, hiatus

hernia and oesophagitis are extremely common because the inhalation of smoke goes from the mouth right down through into the lungs causing all the linings of the inside to get damaged.

Caffeine

Caffeine — one of the most widely used and acceptably of drugs – yet it is a stimulant which is in tea, coffee, soda and some pain killers.

Caffeine raises blood pressure, can give you the shakes, headaches, sleep disorders and can cause anxiety.

There is a mass of further information on www.nida.nif.gov

Fact File F

Sexually Transmitted Diseases

There is no gender or age preference here, STD's can affect as many women as men of all age groups. More than 20 different STDs have been identified, and 13 million men and women are infected each year in the United States. Depending on the disease, the infection can be spread through any type of sexual activity involving the sex organs or the mouth; the infection can also be spread through contact with blood during sexual activity.

- Young people are now more at risk as they are becoming sexually active at a much younger age and are also having sex with different partners of both the opposite gender and the same gender.

- People can pass STDs to sexual partners even if they don't actually have the symptoms; all it needs is a single cell of bacteria to pass, especially to someone who has low immunity.

- Frequently, STDs cause no symptoms, especially in women. The health risks though are very high. Some STDs can cause pelvic infections that may lead to scarring of the reproductive organs, which can result in infertility and increases the chance of cervical cancer.

- STDs can be passed from a mother to her baby before, during, or immediately after birth.

- It is possible, especially if having lots of partners that you can attract more than one type of STD, this will have a massive effect on health and immunity.

Just a quick overview of some of the most common STD's

Gonorrhea

Gonorrhea is one of the most common diseases passed from one person to another during sexual activity.

The overall rate of gonorrhea is now increasing, according to the U.S. Centers for Disease Control and Prevention (CDC). Gonorrhea is the second most commonly reported disease in the United States. The CDC estimates that approximately 700,000 new gonorrheal infections occur yearly in the U.S., only about half of which are reported to the CDC.

More than 5% of people between the ages of 18 and 35 have an infection with gonorrhea that they do not know about. New strains are more easily spread and are resisting treatment even with strong antibiotics.

Chlamydia

Chlamydia is the most common sexually transmitted disease (STD) in the United States.

Among adults, about 5% of the population is estimated to be infected.

Among sexually active adolescent females, about 10% are infected.

Most, especially women, have no symptoms.

Healthy Idol

Chlamydia is an infection caused by the bacterium *Chlamydia trachomatis*.

Genital Herpes

Genital herpes is a common, highly infectious disease. Genital herpes causes blisters or groups of small ulcers (open sores) on and around the genitals in both men and women. It cannot be cured, only controlled.

- Genital herpes is extremely widespread, largely because it is so contagious. Carriers can transmit the disease without having any symptoms themselves of active infection.

- As many as 50 million Americans are infected with genital herpes, with 1 million new infections each year. As many as 80-90% of those infected fail to recognize herpes symptoms or have no symptoms at all.

- The highest rates of infection are seen among the poor, those with less education, those using cocaine, and those with many sexual partners

HIV

HIV infection has now spread to every country in the world and has infected more than 40 million people worldwide as of the end of 2003. More than 1.1 million people in the United States have been infected with HIV.

- HIV causes AIDS. The virus causes the immune system to become compromised and destroys the body's ability to fight infections and certain cancers.

- Sufferers of this deadly condition are not able to fight even the simplest of infections such as a cold because their immunity is so weak, anything they catch is potentially life threatening.
- Anyone who has acquired another STD is potentially at risk of attracting HIV - this is because the body defenses (immune system) is compromised.
- Drug addicts, those who share needles are likely to contract HIV from an infected person as this virus can be acquired through blood, it is also contracted through having sex with an infected person, whether oral, anal or vaginal - the virus will spread through the membranes (skin, inside or outside)

It has also been unfortunate that people have contracted this through no fault of their own by receiving a blood transfusion from an infected person.

Hepatitis (A B C)

Hepatitis is a general term that means inflammation of the liver.

Hepatitis A is found in the stools (faeces) of people with hepatitis A. It is transmitted when a person puts something in his or her mouth that has been contaminated with the faeces of an affected person. The virus can also be spread by eating raw or undercooked shellfish collected from water that has been contaminated by sewage.

People who are infected can start spreading the infection about 1 week after their own exposure. People who do not have symptoms can still spread the virus.

Anyone contracting Hepatitis A will have the

Healthy Idol

ability to overcome this as the liver will completely heal itself. Unlike the following B & C

Hepatitis B is contracted through with an infected person, also semen and saliva which may contain some blood. This is a very infectious disease, sometimes the carrier does not show any signs of sickness but they can transmit it to other people.

The acute phase means that most people will recover completely, if for some reason the situation becomes chronic the infection may never go away and it will cause all manner of other illnesses.

The younger you are when you become infected with the hepatitis B virus, the more likely you are to develop chronic hepatitis B.

The rates of progression to chronic hepatitis B are as follows:

- 90% of infants infected at birth
- 30% of children infected at age 1-5 years
- 6% of people infected after age 5 years
- 5-10% of infected adults

Hepatitis C If the inflammation is not reversed, it becomes ongoing and can cause chronic liver disease, which can be serious or even fatal.

At least 75% of people infected with hepatitis C develop chronic hepatitis C.

If the disease progresses to the point at which the liver begins to fail the only treatment is liver transplantation.

Hepatitis C is an increasing public health concern

in the United States and throughout the world and is one of the most common causes of chronic liver disease in the United States and the most common cause of chronic viral hepatitis

About 4 million people in the United States have antibodies to HCV, meaning they have been infected with the virus at some point; *as many as half of them do not know they have the infection.*

The summary is this:

You WILL contract one or more of these STD's if you are sharing needles to take illegal drugs, having multiple sex partners and not using condoms, men having sex with men and not using condoms, women having sex with an infected person, drinking contaminated water or eating food that has been handled by someone contaminated with the virus.

There is also a possibility that being born to a mother who has the virus means you may get this. Working in care centers, hospitals, institutions means you are more at risk.

The liver is your factory and the body needs it to stay alive. Its most important functions are filtering drugs and toxins out of the blood, storing energy for later use, helping with the absorption of certain nutrients from food, and producing substances that fight infections and control bleeding.

The liver has an incredible ability to heal itself, but it can only heal itself if nothing is damaging it.

Healthy Idol

For further information on STD's

- www.avert.org
- www.until.org
- www.healthfoodsblog.com
- www.cdc.gov

Plus many more sites which I hope will help you to understand the extreme problems caused by contacting a disease of this nature. Play safe and be sensible. Value your health and yourself.

Fact File G

Resources

Eating Disorders, Anorexia/Bulimia

National Eating Disorders Association
603 Stewart Street, Suite 803
Seattle WA 98101
Tel: 800-931-2237

- www.nationaleatingdisorders.org
- info@nationaleatingdisorders.org

NEDA provide information and referrals for support groups and treatment of eating disorders.

National Association of Anorexia Nervosa and Associated Disorders (ANAD)
P.O.Box 7
Highland Park, IL 60035
Tel: 847-831-3438

- www.anad.org
- anad20@aol.com

ANAD is the oldest national nonprofit organization offering free counseling and information. They offer referrals, free of charge to therapists and treatment centers across the United States. A network of support groups is available for sufferers and their families.

Healthy Idol

Sexual Harassment and Abuse

National Child Abuse Hotline
804-422-4453 (800-4-A-CHILD)

- www.childhelp.org

There is a 24 hour helpline for young people and parents with any kind of abuse, sexual, emotional and physical. You do not have to give your name and can speak online to a trained person.

Using the internet is a fantastic resource that would not otherwise be available to you but - please be careful when using the internet as there are "adult only" websites with offensive material. If you have, by mistake, found yourself on such a website, get off the site and do not leave your email address, any credit card information or any other personal information such as age, name and address etc.

Never agree to meet anyone that you have met over the internet on a face to face basis unless you are accompanied but preferably do not meet anyone at all.

If you are upset by any obscene language or are puzzled by something that happens please go to an adult who you trust to help you.

Trisha Stewart

Fact File H

THE GLYCAEMIC INDEX

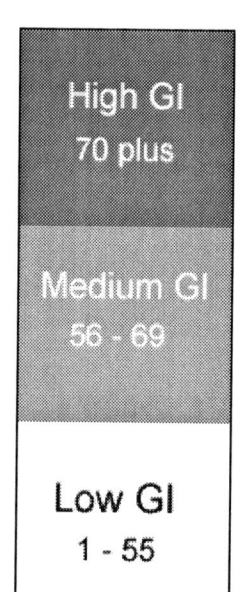

High GI
70 plus

Medium GI
56 - 69

Low GI
1 - 55

The GI or glycaemic index is a system of measuring how different carbohydrate rich foods act on blood sugar levels. A rule of thumb is anything 55 or below because it will act slower therefore sustaining the blood sugar levels.

The GL or glycaemic load is another way of measuring. It lets us know the quality of the carbohydrate. For instance the carbohydrate of the watermelon has a high GI but there is not a lot of carbohydrate in the watermelon so the actual load or GL on the body is low. This means then that the watermelon will spike you up fairly quickly but it will not add too much carbohydrate into your diet.

We'll show more of this on the website as it's another way of working with your food. I'm not too keen on counting either calories or GI/GL but if you're not well, suffering from Diabetes or have other reasons to know what your GI/GL is then it's a good way of monitoring your intake and knowing about both is very useful.

Glycaemic Index (foods selected are based around what we are doing over the 30 days and of course beyond but a more comprehensive index will be available on the website)

Healthy Idol

Food	grams	GI	GL
Whole oats	250	51	11
Pot Barley	150	25	11
Buckwheat	150	54	16
Polenta	150	69	9
Millet	150	71	25
Wholegrain Rice	150	55	18
Rice Noodles	180	61	23
Rice Cakes	25	78	17
Quinoa	65	51	7
Butter beans	150	31	6
Blackeyed beans	150	42	13
Chick peas	150	28	8
Haricot beans	150	38	12
Red Kidney beans	150	28	7
Lentils	150	30	5
Pinto beans	150	39	10
Soya beans	150	18	1
Broad beans	80	79	9
Peas	80	48	3
Pumpkin	80	75	3
Sweetcorn	80	54	9
Beetroot	80	64	5
Carrots	80	47	3

Food	grams	GI	GL
Potatoes (white)	150	88	16 boiled
		85	26 baked
		75	22 fries
		91	18 mashed
Sweet Potato	150	44	11
Swede	150	72	7
Apple	120	38	6
Apricot	120	57	5
Banana	120	52	12
Grapes	120	49	9
Kiwi	120	53	6
Orange	120	42	5
Peach	120	42	5
Pears	120	38	4
Plum	120	39	5
Strawberries	120	40	1
Pineapple	120	66	6
Mango	120	51	8
Grapefruit	120	25	3
Cherries	120	22	3
Watermelon	120	72	4
Hummus	30	6	0
Cashew Nuts	50	22	3